G000016457

Cover illustration by
Richard Moorhouse

RETHINKING REFLEXOLOGY

A new way of looking at an ancient therapy

RETHINKING REFLEXOLOGY

Published by

Douglas Barry Publications

Holborn Gate
1st Floor, 330 High Holborn
London
WC1V 7QT
ENGLAND

Tel 020 7872 5745
Fax 020 7753 2824
E-mail info@DougasBarry.com

FIRST PUBLISHED IN THE U.K. 2003

**RETHINKING
REFLEXOLOGY**

COPYRIGHT 2003
©Douglas Barry Publications

All Rights Reserved. No part of this publication/document may be reproduced or transmitted in any form or by any means, electronic or mechanical, including photocopying, recording, or any information storage or retrieval system, without permission in writing of Douglas Barry Publications.
Written in 2003

British Library - A CIP Catalogue
record for this book is available
from the British Library.

I.S.B.N.   0-9540176-9-2

ACKNOWLEDGEMENTS

To my wife Jean, without whose support this book could not have been written.

To Val and Ray, who have been crucially supportive throughout my venture.

To Margaret Berker, who has given me the encouragement to write this book and helped with the accuracy of the details.

NOTE TO THE READER

This book is not intended as a substitute for professional or medical advice.

Neither the author nor publisher can accept any responsibility whatsoever for any health problem which results from the use of the methods described in this book.

The reader is urged to consult a general medical practitioner as to the cause or nature of a health problem of any sort.

PREFACE

Health bills are rising at an alarming rate and it really is time to find a way of filtering out some of the work and sharing it around alternative ways of achieving desired results without incurring side effects. This will help in reducing the overall expenditure of the nation's health bill.

For this to happen it will need a quantum leap in thought. The impact of what is written here can be enormous if only what is read can be understood. After understanding, comes proof and updating. We have to start somewhere and here is a good place to start.

CONTENT

Chapter 1

Foundations

This book shows Reflexology to its absolute extent. It shows the complexity of how Reflexology interacts with the body to produce healing from within a body's own system. Reflexology in its purest form, as first described by Eunice Ingham and later by Doreen Bailey, works. How it worked was not known; only the knowledge that it did work has been sufficient to justify its existence. This simple fact may be applied to any alternative or complementary therapy. It is true to say that anyone trained in a certain method then goes on to develop that method. I have done this and have developed my own technique. It is this kind of Reflexology that allows the bodily systems to be switched on, to enable the most startling results to become evident.

This book tells of a journey and is a story about how I became a reflexologist. It is probably not too unusual a story, but it is unique to me and therein lies its treasure. I have seen much that others might not on my travels to many different countries. Some of this experience has had a great impact on me, not the least of which is the story about to unfold.

My name is John Moorhouse and I have my own small and private clinic where people of both sexes and all ages attend for treatment. I have seen in excess of 2,000 people for treatment over the last two years. It is from those clients who have attended and are currently attending my clinic that the ideas for this book were derived. In it there may be some things that will be surprising, annoying and hopefully informative.

I like to be honest in my life and I like the public to be treated fairly. There are many different complementary therapies. This is a good thing because what suits one person may not suit another. Most therapists contribute a great deal towards the health of the nation, particularly where the normal medical route has not achieved the desired success. Complementary therapists, in general, try to work alongside the medical authorities, our efforts are often sidelined and thought of as "freaky". Perhaps they think of us with a wizard's or witch's hat, a magic wand and broomstick! The number of people who are now visiting complementary therapists is increasing yearly. So much so, that if the whole of the complementary medical field was shut down tomorrow, the state health organisations would very likely be swamped and grind to a halt.

I have travelled in many countries during my former career in sales engineering and during this activity, much time was spent away from home; time spent waiting at airports sitting on a suitcase, reading a book and waiting for late flights to arrive. When they did, because of the various types of aircraft that were used by different airlines, seating arrangements were varied.

During a long flight, have you ever noticed how people on board an aircraft get up from their seats as soon as the seatbelt signs have gone out ? I used to wonder what they were doing, but gradually, as my back started to ache, the reason became obvious. I started to empathise with them. All this travelling added up to wear and tear on my lower back and pains in my legs. These pains tended to wear off on arrival but when they started to reappear at other times I had to do something about it. Pain killing drugs were taken until the effect that they once had worked no longer. In flight, it was difficult to determine whether or not it was the rattling of the cabin furniture in the aircraft or the pills in my stomach that made the more noise!

On one occasion at home I found that getting up in the morning took longer than normal. My back had become very stiff and took a while to loosen up to the point of comfort. People told me that my body was wearing out! My engineering background told me that any machine will last longer with proper maintenance than without it. There had to be a reason why my back was hurting. Some said that exercise was the answer, but I knew of people who visited the gym two or three times a week and they still had the same problem as me. This state of affairs may well have gone on for years had it not been for a quirk of fate.

On one particular trip to Hong Kong, I was taken by a colleague to an alley way behind a row of restaurants. There we found many Chinese sitting on the kerbstones. These people were all throwing bones and gesticulating with their hands. These people were fortune tellers and, in some cases, it looked as though the information they had given to their customers was unwelcome and payment was being withheld. With the presence of a few "heavies" around it seemed as though any form of resistance was not going to be prolonged. This was not my scene at all.

Having had no previous experience of foretelling the future, the very fact that it was being offered to me was strange and fascinating. The air was heavy with aromas from nearby restaurants and these were mixed with rotting garbage. Vaguely suspicious, I chose a man who had a chair, the only one in the alleyway as far as I could tell. It was odd to think that this small decision was to contribute so much to my future. The man smiled at me, revealing long and very yellow teeth, with one front tooth missing in the upper jaw. He had a long beard but only a few hairs on his chin. He offered to read my hands, face and head. His hands were dark and I could not tell if this was dirt or just skin colouring. The thought of him touching me with those hands was not pleasant. Finally, curiosity overcame scruples and I agreed. The examination of my head involved those horrible hands feeling every detail of my whole head. He went on to examine my sweating palms. After that, he went back to my face. I could smell whatever those hands had been touching before they got to me.

After the hands-on procedure was over he resorted to throwing bones. Well, that did it for me and I was all for leaving but my agent pushed me down and I recovered my composure. The old Chinese man then looked at me and bared those horrible teeth once more: "You will not be doing what you are doing now for much longer, but whatever you do next, you will become a great force in it." I was completely dumbfounded. I paid the man, straightened my clothes, rose from the chair, and left. We travelled back along the way we had come, the hotel room where I was staying now seemed a good place to be after such an encounter. It was easy to be taken in by such a heady mixture of mysticism and all-pervading aromas all of which I could still sense, even after many hours and a long shower. Lying on the bed in the hotel room that night the memory of that evening came to my mind. It was as if this was part of a message, but not having had an experience like this before, it would have been easy to just dismiss it, however I thought that something real was happening to me and I found it very strange. Supposing this man was right and a complete change would occur, what would I do? Where would I go? Soon after returning home to England, the thought that prevailed was the need to stay at home more, the family was growing up and home was where I wanted to be. A Chinese man had said that change was under way, perhaps this was part of a larger message.

Back in the UK my wife and I were visiting a friend's house and discussing complementary medicine, the subject of Reflexology came up. It was something that had come to my mind before but I had taken no action. Perhaps this was a good time to visit a Reflexologist to see if it could help me. To my great surprise and after a comparatively short time, my back problem had eased considerably. During such a visit it was suggested to me that I would make a good Reflexologist if such a course appealed to me. Nothing however could have been farther from my mind, there was an increasing feeling that I needed to be at home much more than in the past. Despite this there was the strange forecast of my future, which involved a change of career. There was a half thought that someone had intimated to me that Reflexology was the way to go. Despite my cynicism even I could recognise that there was indeed a message here and that notice should be taken of its meaning. The required incentive to do something about it eventually came when my last employer and I parted company. The thought gradually dawned that my life had already been mapped out and there should be no need for concern.

My decision was not altogether appreciated at home. There was still the mortgage to pay as well as the bills to be accommodated. The reticence was natural - after all, who had heard about Reflexology? Someone said that it was something to do with tickling the toes, which was degrading as this was my future career. Nonetheless, the die was cast, perhaps my life's experiences would be of benefit to others. It was now with some trepidation that I began to train as a Reflexologist.

Coming from the logical background in engineering sales as I did, the world of Reflexology was a startling change. Instead of dealing with engineering hardware of a specialised nature here I was handling someone's feet. Coming from what was essentially a teamwork situation where everyone in the industry knew everyone else, I found that here you were very much on your own. It was very strange to feel that I was at the starting point, with one foot on the bottom rung of the ladder. I found that most of the trainees were women, all from different backgrounds, each having a unique view on life. It was strange to think that this was the start of something completely new.

It turned out that most of the people who trained on the same course as me were already practising other therapies. Some of these therapies were unknown to me and why they needed other therapies mystified me because, as I saw it, the whole purpose of the training was to create Reflexologists, not multi-therapists. This view was reinforced later when the tutor for the course also expressed reservations about this. The danger was, she said, that during a treatment for Reflexology, other treatments would become part of the session and a mixture of therapies would inevitably take place. This was not to be recommended at all. Some of the trainees simply regarded Reflexology as a useful tool to be added to an existing list of therapies which they already practised. This attitude knocked me back a little and I found it intimidating. These other trainees thought that you must take on other therapies to make a living, however there is not much about client care in that argument. It was clear that those who thought in this way tended to gather together and discuss other therapies, when all we should have been talking about was Reflexology, this after all, was why we were there. Despite this difference of opinion my training progressed and I gained my certificate of qualification in September 1992.

That September, my wife and I set about having a clinic built, attached to my house. That month must have been the wettest on record, or so it seemed. At all stages of the building the rain lashed down. At one stage our kitchen had only three walls, the fourth wall was an open hole where we could watch the rain falling outside and the mud coming in. It was a challenging experience. On the good days it was exciting to see the new building gradually take shape. The builder completed in mid-December and we were left to decorate it in double quick time. I was still laying carpet on Christmas Eve 1992, however, we managed to open on our target date of 2nd January 1993. A chiropractor friend gave me some valuable advice. He once told me that if I stuck like glue to Reflexology then I would become known as a Reflexologist and people would appreciate this and so it proved to be! Here I was, trained, qualified and with my own clinic. It started first with one or two phone calls, which gradually built up over the next two years. The third year was a great success and so it has continued to be ever since.

On completion of my training I became a member of two professional organisations and attended many meetings. At first I found that some people regarded me as different because I was not practising Acupuncture or Aromatherapy or something else in addition to Reflexology. People thought I would not survive. Well, as time has gone on, I have found only a few people who, like myself, practise Reflexology in isolation. I was told, "You get much better results using oils or crystals". This is not so in my experience. I have found that the more you practise Reflexology, the more you learn. One patient's reactions may teach you different things that can be applied to other patients. It is this is knowledge and experience, that comes only from total concentration on the one therapy. My belief is that those who contaminate the Reflexology session with additional appendages only do the therapy a disservice. Reflexology is both a science and a therapy in its own right. Some people, who discuss Reflexology, including many doctors, will say that it is only a way of achieving relaxation. I believe it needs no additions, as the results from Reflexology alone are amazing. By my own insistence and persistence in specialising in Reflexology, I have seen more and more people for treatment, this has allowed me to think more deeply about Reflexology as a healing mechanism and about what happens before, during and after a treatment. I like to think of my progress through this book as a journey. This then is the start of my journey and my thoughts are forming before you, we have a long way to go yet. This book sets out my theories.

Rethinking Reflexology   by   John C F Moorhouse

Chapter 2

Sorting Out

Many books have already been written about Reflexology, and shelves in bookstores dealing with Natural Health matters usually contain many titles. Some books link Reflexology with other therapies, such as Acupuncture or Yoga. There are books relating to pure Reflexology, but they are in the minority. Most of these books are big and attractive, with many showing in detail Reflexology points which correspond to specific parts of the body. These books also show varying Reflexology techniques. Most books will then give case histories where X or Y person has received treatment and amazingly recovered. I could not find one of these books that gave me an insight into how Reflexology works. Some authors have attempted this, but they are still held back by insufficient explanation of the working systems of the body. Most Reflexology books talk a lot about stress, stress patterns and relaxation. This is fine as far as it goes, but even here what we still want to know is how does the whole process of Reflexology work?

I suppose the most significant book written about this subject was by Eunice Ingham. It was she who was the catalyst for Reflexology. Dwight Byers, nephew of Eunice Ingham has been kind enough to furnish me with the following information. Eunice Ingham was a physiotherapist. She practised in the Kirbsville Osteopathic College and Hospital in Kirbsville, Missouri, USA. During the 1930's Eunice Ingham was associated with Dr. Joe S. Riley MD at that hospital and during her time there she became aware of the work done by Dr. William H. Fitzgerald.

Dr. Fitzgerald graduated from the University of Vermont and went on to practise at the Boston City Hospital. Later he travelled to England

and became a member of staff of thé Central London Nose and Throat Hospital. When Dr. Fitzgerald returned to the USA, he took up the position of Head of the Ear, Nose and Throat Department of the St. Francis Hospital, Hartford, Connecticut, USA. It was at this time, Dr. Fitzgerald discovered a Chinese therapy that he renamed and called 'Zone Therapy'. To explain the system he devised the '10 Zone Theory' in which the body is divided into 10 zones running from each finger to the top of the head and then down to each toe. It was claimed by Dr. Fitzgerald and others that treatment in part of a zone would affect everything else in that zone.

Eunice Ingham was a Christian woman and carried those principles into her work. For two years she worked with Dr. Joe S. Riley MD and his wife, who were great followers of Dr. Fitzgerald. During her time with Doctor and Mrs Riley, Eunice Ingham learnt the principles of Zone Therapy and began to formulate her own techniques into what later became known as 'Reflexology'.

According to Dwight Byers, during the late 1930's and 1940's Eunice Ingham brought Reflexology to the attention of osteopaths and chiropractors who were not inclined to pursue it due to the length of time each session would take. It was therefore left to Eunice Ingham to do the pioneering work herself. I wonder if she had any idea of what she was starting. She began to teach her techniques to lay people and semi-professionals. She did this only when she realised that Reflexology was very therapeutic.

In her first book, "Stories Feet Can Tell", Eunice Ingham says how much she owes to Doctor and Mrs Joe S. Riley and it was during her stay with them that she wrote this first book. In her second book, "Stories The Feet Have Told," Eunice Ingham asks for further investigation into Reflexology but what is found in this book adds to the story and pushes it further along the path of knowledge. Eunice

Ingham taught Reflexology to a British nurse who was working in America at the time. Her name was Doreen Bailey and it was she who introduced Reflexology to Great Britain.

Many books can be found about Reflexology, with most giving a similar account of the different authors' theories and the history of the subject. Until now most theories have tended to look alike. Other theories may also be proposed in the future and different countries may bring forth different ideas. Today 'Zone Therapy' has largely been left behind and Reflexology has gone from strength to strength. The growing numbers of practitioners internationally and the ever increasing number patients visiting them is where serious work in the therapy is being done, this testifies to its importance in these countries.

It has been said by some in the field that ancient Chinese and Egyptian practitioners used Reflexology. It is attractive to some people to associate the ancients with Reflexology. For all we know, these ancient pictures may show a ceremony being carried out on people who had long ingrowing toenails! In my opinion this is about as far from Reflexology as keeping goldfish is from deep-sea trawler fishing. So, let us get back to the point. Eunice Ingham gave us Reflexology pure and simple and this is how I like to explore it. I am often asked to give talks on Reflexology and I am happy to do this because this is the way to spread the word. When I have given talks on Reflexology in the past, often towards the end of the talk I sometimes see some blank looks. The truth as I see it sometimes goes against any other ideas that the audience may have previously accepted. and theories that I put forward can sometimes be upsetting to those who practise other therapies. After giving a talk, I usually ask the audience to put up their hands if they have a back problem, naturally, only a few people do. I then ask them all to do a little exercise. This involves standing up from the chair on which they are sitting. The way in which they stand up tells the story.

When those who can be identified as having a back problem are asked to confirm that they have pain or stiffness they readily admit to it, but there seems to be an inbuilt tendency to hide the fact that they have such a difficulty. It is amazing how many people are shown to have a difficulty with the back. Surprise amongst the audience is evident when those who are identified as having a backache reveal that they actually do little or nothing to alleviate their situation.

When asked why they do not try Reflexology, the replies include: "I can't afford it", "not convinced", "have never thought about it", "I am ashamed of my feet" and "why should I pay for it?" At one such meeting a lady said to me that she had a painful backache. "It hurts right across my lower back", she said, indicating the area either side of the sacro iliac joint . The lady went on to say that her doctor was a wonderful man and had given her pills for the pain. It turned out that she had been taking these anonomous pills for thirty years. On enquiry, I found out that she was still taking these pills. " and how was her back now?", "terrible". When told that she should go back to the doctor to review the situation, she repeated, "He is a wonderful man." There was no more to be said. During the intervals I mixed with the audiences as usual and I found that the suspicion was that Reflexology was perceived as some sort of "black magic". Even after a whole evening spent explaining and giving out information nothing could persuade them otherwise. At one particular talk that I gave, I asked for a volunteer with a back problem and one person duly came forward. A treatment was given in accordance with my developing theory and sure enough her back started to get 'warm' (see later in chapter 5). She was pleasantly surprised and even more surprised when I asked her to stand up and she found she could do so with considerably less trouble than before. The audience was appreciative and they were then invited to take part in the same exercise to discover who amongst them had a bad back. I invited each of these sufferers to visit me for treatment. To date no one from that group has taken up the challenge.

I take a philosophical view about this. It is amazing that even when shown the way to achieve a positive result, people are reluctant to do anything about it. Perhaps finance is the main problem, though it is difficult to tell. If it is, then I am sure that by phoning a Reflexologist, a mutually acceptable arrangement can be reached, normally something can be done, an arrangement to ease things along. An arrangement can perhaps be reached whereby the client pays on a structured plan or the client could ask their doctor to provide the necessary finance. Later in this book you will see how I believe that ignoring a stiff or 'bad' back or neck and shoulders can be a real risk for the future.

There is a long way to go to enlighten the public to fully accept that Reflexology can bring such enormous benefits to an individual in a physical sense. Solving many difficulties can also give back to the client the ability to cope with life more easily and this has been seen often in the clients I have treated. Of course the client only feels like a new person, but in reality they are the same person they used to be a long time ago before the problems started. Today Reflexology has spread all over the world and it is appreciated in many countries because it is non-intrusive and there are no side effects. For economically hard pressed countries, it can be of enormous help to the people as no drugs or machines are used. All that is necessary is the skill of the practitioner and a thorough knowledge of human anatomy and physiology.

Worldwide Reflexology is being taught in many different ways. With many cultures taking it on board, we are bound to see it practised differently to the way in which I was trained. We have to accept that the presentation may change but the essence must remain the same. I hope that we, the Reflexologists from wherever we are trained, can all come to realise that variation in training can only enrich the discipline of Reflexology. We must however be careful not to contaminate Reflexology by introducing other therapies and appendages such as crystals and oils etc. With some schools, teaching Reflexology is done in addition to other therapies. Insufficient importance is given to the to the practice of Reflexology, which in my opinion leaves the practitioner inadequately qualified. In its pure form, Reflexology can stand alone and needs nothing to support it. If Reflexology is being used to improve other therapies or if Reflexology is being supported by other appendages, then the 'Reflexologist' concerned is not a good Reflexologist. If a practitioner feels the need to act in such a manner then they should consider doing something else. It is with all this in mind that I have developed my theory of how Reflexology works. I wanted to spread this message to patients and practitioners alike; Reflexology is effective, is a science in itself and there are no negative side effects.

Perhaps I can spend a little time saying something about spiritual help. I have had no contact, of which I am aware, either visual or auditory from within or otherwise, with anyone from the "other side". Having said that, I couldn't account for various events that have changed my life. I treat one person whom I believe is most definitely in contact. She has given me an insight into another world, I cannot deny it and nor would I wish to. I am told of "people" helping me. No direct contact with me has occurred and I have to take this information on trust. All I want to say here is that if I am being helped then I am absolutely delighted. How much of this help directly accounts for the therapeutic effect on the patient is not certain but what I do believe is that the original designer of our bodies, and there surely is one, actually gave us the means to keep us well and happy. It is these same means of healing that the Reflexologist employs. The systems of the body are 'persuaded' into action and it is this action that I find so wonderful and for which I am so grateful. Other people have also given me assurances that I am getting spiritual help and although I cannot report that this is so, I am very happy with the situation.

I want to explain to the reader of this book that I cannot discount any extra help during a Reflexology treatment session but it is without my knowledge. Being a Christian, I have a sneaking suspicion that I am being helped quietly and without fuss, but everyone will have an individual opinion on this. 'Healing' obviously comes to mind when talking about this subject. 'Healing' is another form of treatment and should not be introduced intentionally into the treatment session without the patient's knowledge and agreement. If 'Healing' as a treatment is required then the patient should be referred on to someone who does such treatment. This may sound peculiar in view of my previous words, but in this life Reflexology is one therapy and "Healing" is another. To divorce healing from any therapy may be anathema.

A good thing about Reflexology is that the patient does not have to undress. The fact that no drugs need to be prescribed is also reassuring because it is supposed to be a natural therapy. Only bare feet are required and while we're on this subject, a word should be said for those with ticklish feet. I have come across many with this problem and for the most part, this treatment is able to overcome the feeling and no discomfort is felt. Not everyone with the problem is in this category, but the brave usually appreciate the benefit more than their fear. Most people welcome the comforting experience from one who really knows how to handle feet properly. Those who think that their feet are too awful to be seen should not worry, a Reflexologist will see so many feet and each will display a different appearance; so there is no need to be afraid.

What is not often appreciated should be realised is that feet are every bit as important as any other part of the body. Problems such as fungi, athlete's foot, eczema and other skin ailments should be controlled without delay. The feet deserve it. What they don't deserve is bunions. These happen where the big toe is forced against the second toe. The skin becomes reddened and shiny. After sometime, the bunion becomes painful. In general, bunions are caused simply by forcing feet into badly fitting shoes. The best solution is to wear well fitted (but not necessarily expensive) shoes. Get these shoes from a shop where the people know how to fit shoes properly as experience is everything. The wish to wear fashion shoes is understandable, but even here good fitting is so important. If shoes cause discomfort then good advice might be where those shoes known to be 'pinchy' but unavoidable are taken off at the earliest possible time. At the very least, during the day wear the preferred but 'wrong' shoes for the minimum length of time. The feet will benefit by the toes having an opportunity to realign themselves.

Frequently, feet are presented where the outlines of the toes clearly show the shape of the shoes worn previously or now being worn. Many people blame the shoes they wore in the 1970's and 1980's. It must be stressed that bunions are the result of long term abuse. This is a shame because most bunions are preventable with just a little common sense and thoughtful application. To look after the feet will be in the owner's interest and a more comfortable maturity may be looked forward to. They will also feel nicer. It is true that the feet are a long way down and untouchable to some and we tend to wrap them up in socks, stockings and tights. Then we stuff them into shoes and boots and tend to forget about them, feet deserve more than that. It is precisely because we forget the feet that they become virgin territory for the Reflexologist. Reflexes are more pronounced here than anywhere else on the body and this is why Reflexologists use them as the healing centre. Of course, if through advancing years or disability, it is not possible to use the feet, the hands can also be used.

At the 1995 conference for the Jennifer Trust for Spinal Muscular Atrophy, Reflexologists were invited to attend and give treatment to the carers as well as to the afflicted. All who received treatment were surprised at how they were made to feel better. The look on their faces were clear to see and they said that they would encourage others to take the treatment, when they had returned to their own homes.

It is worth mentioning that those that I treated experienced a feeling of warmth in their legs after the treatment. Their experience was fascinating to me and its significance was not fully recognised until later.

Rethinking Reflexology   by   John C F Moorhouse

Chapter 3

Road to Damascus

The normal accepted route to Reflexology was via Zone Therapy but for me many doubts surrounded the basic premise of artificially dividing the vertical body into ten 'zones'. It just didn't look right and in my opinion this provided uncertainty about the very origins of Reflexology itself. Although this insecurity regarding Reflexology existed in my mind, there was no denying that its benefits to clients were not in doubt. Getting right to the 'hard' expressions in Reflexology so far, let's look at 'energy'. Many people talk about 'energy' when discussing Reflexology, yet nowhere could I find a satisfactory explanation of its meaning in this context. This was surprising to me because so many people discussed it as though it was a matter of fact. I am not referring to energy in the form of electricity as this is not the type of energy often talked about by Reflexologists. It seems to be more of a mystical type. Indeed, the very origin of Reflexology is steeped in 'energy' explanations. Dr. Fitzgerald's Zone Therapy talks about energy running along the ten zones, but for me there were many questions to be answered about these origins.

Coming from an engineering background this type of thinking was very hard to accept. I remember being at a seminar for Reflexologists where the speaker was freely talking about 'energy'. I listened for a long time and then asked what the speaker meant by energy, no positive answer was forthcoming. Instead, the speaker asked those present if anyone in the audience could give me an explanation but once again, none was forthcoming. It was therefore clear that I was not the only one who had difficulty in understanding what was meant by 'energy'. There had to be a more rational explanation of energy in Reflexology.

In 1992 it was announced that during the following year there would be a European Conference on Reflexology and it would be held at the University of Newcastle-upon-Tyne, U.K. As I live and breathe Reflexology, and it is part of my life, this was not an opportunity to be missed as this was the first such event in Europe. Upon arrival at Newcastle University I soon began talking with other delegates. There we were, all waiting with keen anticipation.

Attending this conference were Reflexologists from all over the UK and Ireland plus many others from a wide range of countries. It was fascinating to hear the thoughts of all those people as the papers were presented to packed audiences.One paper was entitled "An Holographic Approach to Reflexology", by Helle Johanneson of Denmark. She had been commissioned by the Danish Reflexologists Association (Forenede Danske Zoneterapeuter - F.D.Z.), to find an approach as to how Reflexology works through the work that she was doing with holographic photography. After settling some details with the FDZ she agreed and set to work. With my background in engineering, the subject she had chosen, on paper, looked interesting to me. We all went into the main conference hall and sat down. The usual hubbub of pre-lecture noise was higher than usual. At last the hall was brought to quiet and the speaker was introduced.

When Helle Johannesson took the floor (at first sight) she did not appear as I expected. She spoke of her work in almost perfect English and this was such a compliment to us. As she got into her speech I could see some around me fidgeting and even blinking their eyelids. For me on the other hand, what was being said was the most amazing thing I had heard for a very long time. It was like a door opening and a light suddenly filling my mind. At last I was beginning to see properly. With the kind permission of Halle Johannesson, here is a shortened version of the paper she presented at the Newcastle-upon-Tyne conference.

"Holography is the name of a new kind of three-dimensional picture, used for photographing museum pieces, medical examinations, developing new forms of transportation, as well as creating new works of art.

Holography is also a new scientific way of perceiving the world, and the holographic principle is predicted to greatly expand future scientific work. An important aspect of holography is: *THE PART REFLECTS THE WHOLE.* This principle may, therefore, explain the existence of reflex zones in the feet and the fact that there is an effect in the body when the feet are treated. It may also explain the effects of other complementary therapies built on the idea of the part reflecting the whole. Using a map of the feet with a projection of the entire body, Reflexology is based on the principle of the part reflecting the whole. Until now, it has been difficult to explain the connection between the feet and the rest of the body, since no direct link between reflex zones and the corresponding organs has been found.

Using a holographic way of thinking, this problem solves itself, because holography is not built on ideas of mechanical and direct connections between part and whole. In a holographic model of Reflexology, the issue is not finding a direct link between, for example, the liver and the zone.

The connection is structural and consists of a correlation between the pattern of the feet and the overall pattern of the body. The feet and the body are both interpreted as an expression of a common organising pattern for this particular individual. When manipulating the pattern in the feet the common organising pattern is altered, thereby influencing the pattern in the entire body. The principle of holography is not limited to describing the relationship between feet and body. It includes relations between the body as a whole and various body-parts, such as anatomical parts, ears, eyes, etc. - and different dimensions, such as the biochemistry of the body, psychological factors, etc. Feet and ears, biochemistry and psyche can be regarded as different expressions of the organising pattern of the patient. Many different approaches to treatment of the individual human being therefore exist.

On the other hand, the health problems experienced by the client have many possible explanations, i.e. anatomical, biochemical and/or psychological, each of which supplements the other in our understanding of the complicated being each client represents. In a broader perspective, the holographic principle illustrates the client and the therapist as conscious, sensing and acting beings in the same (holographic) world. Reflexology, acupuncture of the ear, placebo effects and others, so far inexplicable phenomena, may thus become quite logical within scientific frames of reference.

In the light of all this, it may be worth to considering the use of the holographic explanation as part of an attempt to obtain "official recognition of Reflexology."

There was a lot more, but that was enough for me. Well, I could not presume to liken myself to St Paul, but if ever someone else had had a 'Road to Damascus' experience, this was certainly mine. When she was finished I felt as though like I had been washed through on the inside. She left the stage but I felt that I wanted to continue so we could brainstorm our way through this. Unfortunately, the pressure of the programme prevented us from continuation. On looking at other delegates after the paper had been delivered, I expected to see faces full of similar amazement, but I did not see any. We sat through the rest of the conference programme and the delegates applauded. For me however, the conference had already ended. At the actual finish of the conference as we all said our goodbyes and went our separate ways, I was still amazed at what I had heard from Halle Johannesson. The suggested explanation of the relationship between the feet and the rest of the body had already started to embed itself into my mind and my brain was working overtime. If every cell has DNA, which we know to be true, then we also know that DNA is the building structure for the whole body. As the body grows and changes then the information in the cell also changes.

For example, my nose as it was when I was a baby is quite different to the nose that I now have now as an adult. If I damage my nose it will be repaired, as it should, to its condition now; not as it was when I was a baby. Also, the position of my nose must be accounted for in relation to my eyes and ears. It must look right (if ever it can look right!) in relation to the rest of my body. The DNA in a single cell is the basis for the whole body and so if the information in the single cell is to be current about my nose, then it must contain current information about the rest of the body. That information applies not only to the structure of the body, but also about the condition of the body. If Helle Johanneson's paper is correct then the amount of information in a single cell is not as detailed as is that which would be contained in a larger group of cells collectively. When more and more cells group together, then the current information about the entire body in that group of cells becomes clearer and more detailed.

It is rather like viewing a distant object through a telescope. It is not possible to see the fine detail of the object at a great distance. When, however, the object draws nearer, more details of it become visible. The nearer it gets, the greater the detail which can be seen, until, when the object is standing next to you no telescope is needed and every detail is visible.

In perspective then, in the case of Reflexology, the information in a large group of cells, i.e. the feet, contains some detail but not all. This information is enough for the condition of the various organs and limbs in the body to be identified on the feet. Hence if this information is a representation of the body, then there has to be a recognition of that representation by the brain and a connection made between the feet and the actual position in the body itself. If the group of cells, (as in the case of Reflexology we take the feet), contain information about the geographic position of each organ etc., then they must also contain information about the condition of each organ. Either good, bad or somewhere in between. I call this *INTERCELLULAR* information and the pain on the feet related to the corresponding body position, *INTERCELLULAR* pain. If the intercellular information contained in the feet is current, then it is quantitatively and qualitatively descriptive of the status of the body's age, wrinkles and pain. This intercellular information relates to the current condition of the body. When there is a problem in a particular part of the body, the deviation from the norm (see chapter 5), is exhibited as intercellular pain. The appropriate position on the foot, where the client experiences pain, is registered by the brain which uses the information in the cell structure to co-relate it to the actual position in the body where the injury site is. This intercellular pain is not indicative of the condition of the feet themselves but is the giving up of the information held in the cell structure. Not only that, the pain felt by the client can be interpreted by the experienced Reflexologist as an indication of a nerve problem or muscle pain. If a reflex point on the feet is active, it gives up this intercellular information and converts it into pain, this pain passes into the neural network and is felt by the client. This pain is registered by the client's brain, with the result being that they say "ouch". I have been kicked on some occasions where the client has reacted in response to the intercellular pain, of course the client is not aware of what is happening, they only feel pain.

The intercellular pain in the feet is felt because of the connection to the brain through the neural network. There is of course a connection because the legs work, and they work because of instruction from the brain and so the connection is made. The picture of the body, in a little detail, as represented on the feet, is recognised by the brain. This is true as will be demonstrated later in this book. The means of connection has to be through the neural network, as there is no other route. As the brain knows all, sees all and does all, it achieves all through the neural network. The nervous system is the eyes of that part of the brain which monitors the day to day condition of the body. The staggering importance of the brain and the neural network is becoming clearer.

Up to this point then, through deduction, we have established that there is a connection between the brain and the intercellular pain in the feet over and above the normal connection foot pains that a client might experience during everyday living. The brain puts the information incoming via the neural network through its monitoring function, into every cell in the body. This operation is constantly updating the quality and severity of the pain experienced by the client. The intercellular pain on the feet, called reflex points, also varies in style (sharp, bruising, sore, etc.) and severity. A severe pain in the neck shows up as a severe pain in the foot, a slight pain in the neck shows up as a slight pain in the foot. The pain experienced by the client is registered by the brain in response to the information coming through the neural network. The pain felt by the client is directly proportional to the severity of the condition. Likewise, the pain felt in the foot is directly proportional to the pain in the neck.

I am aware of the 'Gaia Theory', formulated by James Lovelock. This theory involves, amongst others, the relationship between the earth and its components. An event in one part of its structure and a balance event in another part of the earth, affects the entire earth. There is a lot more to this but the above essence is enough for us to see a similarity in the Gaia Theory, where it is thought that there is a mass consciousness all over the world. A person in America might make a discovery on a Tuesday and another person, for instance in

Sweden, announces the same discovery on Wednesday. The Gaia Theory suggests that there is a link between the two events and they are part of the mass consciousness, which makes both sets of people have similar thoughts. There is a similarity between the essence of the Gaia Theory and my theory of the cells of the body having the same information as every other cell. It is an interesting thought.

The feet are a very large grouping of cells therefore it is possible to make this information clearer in a representative form. It is quite possible therefore that if a client has a neck problem and absolutely nothing else wrong in their body, the only pain felt on the feet will be on the big toe of each foot. Likewise, if there is nothing wrong with the client at all, there will be no pain on the feet. Because the grouping of cells on the feet is relatively large it is not difficult to extend this idea to expanding the detail more and splitting the body into two equal parts vertically. Thus one half of the body is represented by the one foot on the same side. It is now possible to establish that the neck pain may be on, say, the left side of the neck only, because the pain in the feet is on the left foot on the big toe only. It is not possible to say exactly what is wrong in any greater detail, such as glaucoma in the eyes, infection, conjunctivitis or anything else. Only the client can clarify further. The brain sees only the fact that there is a problem and not what specific problem it is, according to the labels that we give to different indications. (See chapter 5 - Lifepath Theory)

We can appreciate then that there is a live connection between the feet and the brain through the neural network. There is a relationship between the feet and the rest of the body. There is a relationship between the pain in the body and pain in the feet. We are on our way!

So, as Reflexologists we work with feet. Up to now, all we had was Zone Therapy, but now, here is a radical new look at the basis of Reflexology. Here seems to be an acceptable attempt at an explanation of the relationship between the feet and the rest of the body in Reflexological terms. At last we are getting out of the mystical area and getting into realism. The brain knows all, therefore if a person has a pain in the right shoulder joint, they are well aware of where the pain is because it hurts. The brain is also well aware of the intensity and the location of the problem. What we have not appreciated before is that the rest of the body is also aware of the problem, so when the reflex area for the right shoulder on the foot is given specific pressure, the person says "Ouch!". Here, then, is the connection. The brain recognizes the reflex area on the right foot as the corresponding right shoulder on the body.

Here I had followed the thinking behind the approach by Halle Johannesson and extended it. This was only the start and what I needed to do was to continue along these lines. I searched through all the books that I could lay my hands on about Reflexology and nowhere could I find a satisfactory explanation of how the therapy actually works. As stated before in this book I could find no satisfactory explanation of what some Reflexologists call 'energy'. What was needed now was a real look at what was going on. I hope that this may be answered in the next few chapters.

Chapter 4

The Push Forward

There is a reason for everything. Drawing on my own observation and experience, I found that by listening properly to what a patient is telling you, most of the clues come from them at the time of the consultation and treatment. There has to be a reason why things go wrong. All the cases in the following pages of Chapter 4 are based upon work and observation carried out in my own clinic.

I have started on my journey and am I getting a little nearer to my goal? Well, maybe; that is the putting down of my thoughts into a workable theory which will take me further along the road. Following on from Chapter 3, I decided to clarify my own objectives and devise a work pattern to further my thoughts about the healing process. I had often heard my patients tell me that after treatment they experienced a feeling of warmth in the area of pain. It was this phenomenon that was of interest to me and it needed to be explored further. To keep it simple and in order to explain what I found, we will keep to one example through the next section.

Many people who come to me complain of lower back pain. Their ages vary from twenty-seven to seventy-two years, and they are mostly women. The common reflex area to all these patients was that representing the sciatic nerves. I decided to look at thirty patients with lower back pain and, with their agreement, began treatment of the sciatic loop reflex area in combination with isolation treatment to the sacrum spine, sacro-iliac joint and pituitary gland only. In each case, the reflex area for the sciatic nerve was painful, in some instances very painful. Treatment to the sacrum spine, sacro iliac joint, sciatic nerves and pituitary gland was given later, to the exclusion of all else. Pressure was maintained on the sciatic nerve reflexes for a three and a quarter minutes period and then released. The pain in the reflex point on the feet went from being hurtful to being numb and then free of pain altogether. After a short time many patients started to experience 'tingling' in their lower back area. This happened fairly quickly and although the time varied from patient to patient, it was in the region of thirty seconds to three minutes. I have known other patients who take much longer. This tingling was in fact in the same area as the injury site that was giving the pain. Soon, the tingling subsided, perhaps after thirty seconds to one minute. There then followed an increasing feeling of 'warmth'. This was around the same injury site in the lower back and was described as being like a glow or warmth. Occasionally, it became very hot. If the original pain in the lower back had been intense then sometimes a 'throbbing or pulsing' was experienced. This glow gradually transformed into a general feeling of warmth and then spread over the whole of the lower back, buttocks and legs. This warmth stayed in the pain site and the rest of the legs, as above, until the end of the treatment session, usually forty-five minutes, when it would start to reduce in intensity. For some it was found that the feeling of warmth often stayed with them after they had left the clinic. In all cases it was found that there had been a significant reduction of pain by the end of the session.

People treated	Complaint	Age	Sex	Effects and results
6	Lower back	40ish	Male	Back pain reducing to heat then cooling and finally relief.
20	Lower back and leg pains	45ish	Female	A lot of tingling in lower back and legs turning to heat then to warmth. Result relief.
6	Lower back	45ish	Male	Heat in whole trunk & shoulders then turning to warmth. Relief was felt.

LET'S LOOK AT THE TABLE ....

I began to consider what was going on here. The evidence I had gathered started to gel in my mind and I wondered how the information in Chapter 3 played a part in this event. I thought about other occasions where warmth, (in this context), was also experienced.

My mind was taken back to my childhood when I was always banging and hurting myself on furniture, gates, posts and the like. I recalled such an event when my arm had been badly bruised by the contact with a carriage door on a railway train, the pain was so bad that tears flowed and I remember it even now. Following the pain, I saw a dark red area appearing where it hurt, there then followed a change in colour to a darker shade of red, which was followed by a throbbing sensation that gradually subsided. I also remember a feeling of warmth, which after a short time became hot in the injury site 'hurt' area. After a while the pain level reduced and the tears dried up. Of course, now that I am older, the other details are less clear but what I had experienced then reminded me of what had happened to my patients. This was not a million miles away from what my patients were now reporting to me. Could the two events be connected?

Reflexology is my life and everything I do is from that perspective. I try to make the language used in this book simple without too much technical jargon. When one reads some of the current medical literature and magazines, the language used can be difficult to understand. I think this is a problem, as our health is a concern for all of us and the technical language used can often create a barrier. Because of this, we are seeing and hearing people on television, radio or in newspapers from strange sounding medical departments talking about projects at a molecular level and giving explanations of their work, this can be a bit confusing. We all need doctors, hospitals and other institutions, but we may still have difficulty in understanding what is going on. We need them and the pharmaceutical companies to defeat the seemingly endless list of diseases, but let's not forget the public's need for understanding.

I believe that this is one reason why books related to complementary medicine have sold so well. More and more are now available but the important factor is that most are written in clear language without too much jargon. I accept that anatomy and physiology have to have common language worldwide, but I sometimes hear representatives from the medical field talking what I call "MEDISPEAK" and it is very difficult to understand exactly what is being said. All specialist fields have their vocabulary which is used internally, but the interface with the public should be understandable. In other words, the purchasers of such books (who may have no medical training at all) should be able to actually read and understand what they see.

We have moved too far along the allopathic road where people seem to demand a pill for everything. Well these are not always available! The growth of complementary medicine bears witness to customer preference and the demand for help with many different health problems. In the past, the main thrust for alternative treatments came from those people with 'difficult' problems, such as cancer and AIDS. This came about only because people believed that 'normal' allopathic medicine was not getting anywhere, or where the treatment offered was just too awful to contemplate. The body is a delicately balanced living organism and yet within that delicacy comes a powerful ability which copes with accidents, war, pollution, viruses and disease. Tragic or unfortunate as these circumstances are, the body learns to resist or live with them, although it must be said that many people are lucky enough never to experience them. However, what people do often get is backache, knee and elbow pains, migraines, menstrual problems and lumps. Doctors' surgeries are littered with people suffering from these sometimes debilitating complaints. Now we are seeing problems like backache, cystitis, sciatica, migraine and many others being accommodated by the complementary disciplines.

Many people have been struck down suddenly with back pain having done nothing more than get out of bed, turn around in the car or simply having sneezed. Climbing over a gate is not an uncommon cause. How many surgical operations have been carried out in an effort to relieve the pain without success?. It is possible that a vertebra has moved to pinch a nerve, perhaps the sciatic nerves, or maybe some inflammation on the nerve itself suddenly causes the muscles to lock. (I have seen in my clinic that if a patient has a tendency to cramp in the legs, treatment to the sciatic nerves reflexes is a sure way of keeping cramp away.)

All this means more business for the health industry, but misery and pain for the individual, with time off work and the possibility of loss of earnings. How many working hours are lost over this one problem? Many millions I would guess. The same may be said about menstrual problems or migraine. The cost to the sufferer, the employer, the health care system, social services and the nation is enormous. The normal route for a problem such as back pain may be first to see a doctor, whose normal advice, so my patients tell me, might be prescribing pain killers and rest. This can take as much as three to six weeks to complete and so already the costs are mounting up. Next is probably physiotherapy treatment, which will often consist of two treatment blocks with each block consisting of six sessions each. If this is not successful then a visit to the local pain clinic is arranged and epidural injections and additional drug therapies are used. If all fails then surgery is offered without any guarantee of final success. Does this sound familiar ? Please read on and let me tell you about one of my patients.

A lady came to me after having had three operations on the vertebrae of the lumbar region of her spine. The problem originally occurred when she climbed over a five bar gate. The resultant searing pain in her lower back and left leg caused her to see her doctor. Even after three operations on her lower back to stop the pain, it had not subsided. This lady had been through the procedure of taking pills, rest and physiotherapy, culminating in surgery and none of this had helped with the pain. Not unnaturally, she was very worried that she might remain like that for the rest of her life. This was when she was advised by a friend to see a Reflexologist.

This was her first encounter with complementary therapy and so understandably, she was apprehensive about seeing me. Her husband came into the treatment room with her, and they talked to each other during this first session. This is not something I usually encourage but, in such cases, it is necessary. Treatment was given to the whole spine, sciatic nerves and sacro-iliac joint. Even after the first treatment she obtained substantial relief. She reported that she felt a deep warm sensation in her lower back and both legs, reaching down to her feet and this happened at every subsequent treatment. She said that she could not believe that the relief enjoyed could be possible after just one treatment. She had been enjoying the week without the pain but would not chance anything that might upset things. On that first visit and subsequent visits, she felt this deep warmth. This was understandable but it did seem that a significant event had occurred which appeared to be the healing process in progress. Subsequent visits reduced her pain level to just about zero. On each occasion she felt the warmth in the lumber region of the spine, in her buttocks and in both legs. With treatment running into six weeks we began to see the intensity of the heat reduce and this corresponded with the report from the patient that she was feeling 90% better. I concluded that she was now able to go on holiday with confidence, decorate her house, do the gardening and perhaps best of all, she could now lift her grandchildren without worry. Undoubtedly she was now experiencing a much better quality of life. Once again the sciatic nerve reflexes on the feet had represented the principal painful areas in the body. It seemed that the sciatic nerve, this being the only connection between the lumbar spine and the toes, had been in trouble and this condition had responded very well to the treatments. Later, we found that the healing process was still present but in the right hip and the right thigh. The patient reported that she had got total relief from the chronic back pain with which she had first presented, but we could not totally shift the right hip problem. I have since established that the patient has returned to the doctor where a CT scan has shown osteoarthritis. It was clear that the problem in the hip area had unfortunately gone too far before she came to me for treatment.

This sort of result cries out for an explanation. What had happened to bring about this dramatic change? Had the gentle but persuasive treatment of the relevant reflex areas on the feet brought about such a tremendous change? I decided to see if this sort of result could be repeated over more people with various problems, not just backache. A few examples follow:

A lady came to me with pain in her right ear. She had been to see her doctor who had not offered a real diagnosis but had thought there may be an inflammation in the ear. Antibiotics had not cleared the problem and painkillers were the only help. She was experiencing noises in the ear and was naturally concerned. I treated the ear reflex with firm but not harsh pressure. She felt pain (like a bruise) at the reflex area on the right foot, and also the reflexes for the cervical spine, neck and shoulder on the big toe and across first joints between the distal phalanges on the top of the right foot. Constant pressure was applied to each of the above reflex areas for a total of three minutes. We then waited for any change. Sure enough, she started to feel tingling in the cervical spine and shoulders and the outer ear. This tingling then turned to warmth after a few seconds, which then lasted about fifteen seconds. Not only that, the warmth was travelling into the inner ear where it stayed warm for some twenty minutes more.

The pain started to gradually reduce after ten minutes into the twenty minute warm time. The noises in the ear were erratic. At the end of twenty minutes the warmth began to rapidly reduce and finally faded altogether. Even though her ears were not totally pain free, the noises were reduced.

The lady came back for three more treatments and each time the same thing happened. During the last session the warmth was not present at all, it had been reducing in intensity with each session, but as there was now no warmth at all I believe that it meant that no more healing needed to be done. The lady had felt improvement week by week and was not now not troubled by either pain or noises in her right ear. She was delighted with her good fortune and also that she had no more need of painkillers. I repeated this type of treatment, as a form of clinical research, to a further twenty people, to support my theory, which was beginning to take shape. The object would be to establish the effect on presented problems by using Reflexology on the feet and by applying treatment to the reflexes relevant to the injury site, allowing observation of the resulting effects which were executed by the body's own internal systems following treatment. In each case the patient exhibited similar indications, cold feet, knees hurting, kneecaps clicking, ankles clicking and cramp. Those with long-term back pain/stiffness also had varicose veins.

It is worth considering the following example, which illustrates the above clearly. A lady who had a diagnosed problem with her bladder came to see me. She had been told that she had got a lazy sphincter muscle and was consequently suffering inadvertent leakage of urine. She did not know if it was the inner or outer muscle. She was having to wear incontinence underwear to cope with the problem. An operation was offered but she was uneasy about such surgery, so had refused. Instead, a friend recommended that she should come to see me. She came and agreed to my research proposal. During the first session she was totally surprised to find that her feet did not feel ticklish during the treatment as she thought they would.

She had stressed that her feet were normally very sensitive. The reflex areas on the feet for the bladder, lumbar-sacrum, coccyx spine, sciatic nerve and pituitary gland on both feet were located and treatment was applied in a gentle but firm manner for a total of three minutes. The lady found that the feeling was similar to that of pressing on a bruise which was uncomfortable, but not unbearable. After one minute she reported that the pain on her right foot started to fade. After two minutes the pain was no longer evident, it had gone completely. I carried on for the third minute and then released the pressure. The same treatment was then repeated on the left foot. The same pattern was followed with pressure released after the third minute. In order that we could both see what changes might be produced by that treatment, we both relaxed and waited for something to happen. I explained that I had expected her to feel tingling and/or warmth in her groin. After another five minutes the lady said she could feel tingling in her lower abdomen and groin, her lower back also felt tingly. A few minutes later she said she could feel these tingly areas turning warm (she said glowy). At first she felt tingling and warmth together and then she reported that the feeling of warmth was 'overcoming' the tingly feeling until the tingling finally subsided. She remained warm but then felt heat in her groin, she said that she felt this event in the lower back first then it 'spread' over the whole of the lower back and then into the abdomen. She said, "I can actually feel warmth inside my groin." The whole of the pelvic floor was warm by this time. This effect continued for another twenty minutes and then the warmth began to 'cool off'. When she was only slightly warm, she visited the toilet and then we discussed what had happened. She was quite happy and went home.

The same lady returned the following week, she reported that no positive effect had been experienced on her bladder. In fact, her condition was a little worse. However, her backache, she was pleased to report, was much better. Back ache! What backache? This had not been revealed earlier, although the warmth in her lower back should have alerted me to it.

The second session started with the same treatment pattern being applied to both feet as before. The reflex areas for the bladder proved to be less painful than they were the previous week and this time, the bladder reflexes cleared of pain very quickly. After only one minute she felt warmth in her groin and lower abdomen, her lower back was also warmed. Treatment ceased for the right foot and pressure was released from the right foot after one minute and the same on the left. By the time pressure was applied to the left foot her lower abdomen was already warm. She reported feeling the warmth without any tingling this time and she said that the tops of her thighs also felt warm; she had no explanation for this but I was beginning to see some pattern. The warmth cleared after twenty minutes and by this time she was beginning to enjoy the experience. She was certainly more comfortable than when she had arrived. She used the toilet and left.

The following week, she returned with a big smile. She told me that no leakage of urine had occurred at all during that week and she had felt confident enough to start wearing ordinary underwear. She was delighted. Treatment was continued as before but no pain was felt on the bladder reflexes. Warmth was still felt in the lower abdomen only but the feeling was slight. At the end of the session she left without visiting the toilet.

The following week the lady reported no further problem. There was no pain on either foot at the relevant reflexes and no warmth was experienced in her body. At the end of the session, she and I concluded that something remarkable but natural had happened and this warmth was obviously the key.

On another occasion, I was treating a man who had lower back pain and he too experienced the warmth. He said he thought it was not possible to experience such heat without using a heating element and he was amazed. What does all this tell me? Something was going on but there was no explanation yet. As I have said before in earlier chapters, I could have just left it there and just accepted it. Many therapists have told me that the warmth is of a mystical 'energy' but none could define it. I could not accept that because I believe that the miracle is in us. We are the miracle. Whoever designed us or however we arrived here on earth, our bodies were given the means to keep us alive and well and in a comfortable condition from birth until death. I felt that any strange happening, such as the warm feeling that patients were telling me about, should be regarded as the result of a natural reaction in progress.

Well, what was I to make of the results? I could have just left it there and told other Reflexologists about what had happened. I could have compartmentalised the information and accepted it as a supernatural intervention, as some other therapists had done, but I could not leave it there. To the clients who provided me with my results, I say thank you and they can rest assured that they have made a contribution to the further understanding of the reactions which make Reflexology work. The sensation of warmth that was experienced by my clients was the common manifestation in all treatments and this was to be the focus of my thoughts.

So what had I got up to this point? Had Halle Johannesson's paper at Newcastle sought to propose a possible link between the reflexes on the feet and the rest of the anatomical parts of the body, through her work with holographic photography? I had also got the anecdotal evidence from the specific treatments given to patients, which provided the reports of the common effect of the 'warmth'. Of course, this common link seemed to be very valuable evidence. I have developed a new way of delivering Reflexology, which I call 'Neuroflexology' (Reflexology at the second level). All treatments hereafter and their results are given with R2. I have also found new areas on the feet that give faster and more positive recovery.

The conclusion of these treatments must mean that the body has responded to treatment of the relevant reflexes in the feet, which corresponded to the injury site(s) in the body. This has been regarded by the brain as a friendly instruction, the body systems have reacted positively and the healing process has been initiated. It is the healing process that has created the beneficial effect on the patient to a greater or lesser degree, depending on the severity of the presented symptom.

Something happens after Reflexology treatment is given. Is the warmth the 'energy' (whatever that is), that some therapists talk about, or is there another event in progress?

Chapter 5

The Theories

So my journey to wherever I am going has progressed ever further. From a position where I had only thoughts, to where I am presently, building these thoughts into facts. Now answers are needed. Everyone in the business of health should have the aim of making the patient's life more comfortable and to improve his or her quality of life. This falls to Reflexologists as well as doctors. The trouble is that doctors do not understand Reflexology and yet neither do many Reflexologists. Before we get into the theories themselves, it should be understood that I classify the 'diseases' of the human body into two basic categories: internal diseases and external diseases. Internal diseases are those that occur in and maybe are generated within the body, without outside influences. These may occur after many years remaining undetected. Included in this category are osteoarthritis, breast lumps, migraine, cold feet, prolapsed organs, enlarged organs, heart and vascular circulation problems (blood pressure). The external diseases are those that are impacted upon the human body by outside forces and substances, such as chicken pox and other viruses, war, violence, accidents and pollution. There is a huge difference between the two and in this book I will be dealing only with what I call internal diseases.

During the course of this chapter the importance of the brain in all matters of health becomes obvious and paramount. Since I have looked at the human body in this way, my perception of it has been changed and as a result I began to visualise the body stripped away to reveal the brain and neural distribution system in isolation. The extent of the distribution of the neural network would be incredible. The brain is a highly complex organ, with definitive descriptions of it to be found in many anatomical and physiological books, with most of them written by eminent authors. The study of the brain and nervous system is called Neurology. It serves no purpose repeating here any such description because it would take this book into another area and away from the theory. That the brain is central to our very existence there is no doubt, it is the originator of thought and instruction and it is from there that everything in the body is controlled and monitored. Not just the things with which we normally associate the brain with such as seeing, smelling, touching, hearing, moving, and so on, but also with the normal maintenance of the body. It is clear to me that the body cannot look after itself divorced from the brain. The brain must also be responsible for the maintenance and repair systems so thoughtfully provided for the purpose of keeping us well and comfortable until a natural end. To do this, the brain needs to extract information from the body and monitor its current state against a standard.

There must be a standard or blueprint against which, the body's performance can be checked. If this was not so, then the corrective action taken by the repair systems within the body would go on and on without limit. The brain has a comprehensive standard to compare what is and what should be. This is the benchmark for an individual's comfort and well-being and this standard must provide the parameters within which everything must operate. An illustration would be the liver, prostate or even the heart, all of which are glands/muscles. All have nerves that lead to them and of course are in contact with the brain. Why would this be so? I believe that the standard within the brain is providing the parameters within which they must work and co-habit. This gives, amongst other things, the size that each must be and its geographical position in relation to its surroundings. The brain sees what is going on via the neural network and so it is not unreasonable to conclude that an unimpeaded flow of information from the brain is essential for good health. Of course the brain also contains the thought processes and emotions that can alter the state of the body. However, this is the subject of far greater literature and will not be touched here.

The brain has all this ability to give instructions and receive information through the neural distribution network. This network is a staggering mass of nerves forming a distribution system. Each nerve has a complex construction and each carries exceedingly complex and rapid information back and forth from the brain to the appropriate target, which, for instance, could be a muscle. We divide even the neural network into anatomical sub-divisions, such as the peripheral nerves and the autonomic nerves.

The autonomic nerve system is responsible for the control of bodily functions such as regular heartbeat, digestive system, sweat glands and much more. All these functions operate constantly but we are normally blissfully unaware of their activity and we cannot control the parts of the body to which the nerves of the autonomic system are attached.

Even these autonomic nerves are split again into sub-divisions of sympathetic and parasympathetic systems. Descriptions of the functions of these systems are found in good anatomy and physiology books. The flow of information from the brain to an organ is extremely complex and needs a lot of understanding but we must not limit this complexity to just a purely functional status, there is also a need factor, a need to bring the body back to a standard and to repair a break in the skin until it matches the surrounding tissue. This need is also a hunter, and it wants to regain control in circumstances such as after loss of control through a stroke or perhaps an interruption caused by a breakage of a nerve after an accident. It is difficult to keep thinking of the mass of complexity of the nerve activity and the need factor separately so I will call this whole process "*NEUROFLOW*", this is the flow of information to and from the brain along a nerve. This explanation is in the simplest of terms, but for the purposes of this book it is sufficient. The very fact that we exist at all as a living, moving being is all due to the brain and the *NEUROFLOW*.

An analogy would be that you are at a house and the main door is shut. There is a doorbell but you need to open the door to enter the house and the way in which you can achieve this is to push the doorbell with your finger. As soon as you action the desire the doorbell rings and your ears tell you the bell is ringing, the door does not open so you keep ringing until the desired result is achieved. Your eyes tell you that the door is open so you stop ringing the bell with your finger and in you go.

The means of achieving and satisfying the overall desire was to ring the bell until the door was opened. In this case the desire to enter the house was the standard, the finger on the bell was the instruction and the electrical current was the neuroflow. The ringing of the bell was the work being carried out in pursuance of the need to achieve the desire or standard. So everything that moves or lives within the body owes its very existence and performance to the brain and if the brain really does control everything in the body then perhaps we can extend our thoughts into body maintenance.

How is it that our muscles stay supple and the skeletal joints move without pain? How is it that the production of smooth cells in frictionless lubricant continues to be supplied to joints, only to be washed away after their useful life is over, thus enabling the joint to perform correctly? What does the brain do for the circulation system? After all it does affect the heart. If I extend my thoughts a little further I can surmise that the body as a whole therefore has no intelligence in itself and is entirely dependent upon the brain's intelligence and what it is told to do by the brain. The body can therefore be seen as an extension of the brain, designed to serve the brain itself in its desires and wishes.

Never before have I thought of the whole body as being an entity in this way. In the past I have always thought of a pain in the knee as no more than a pain in the knee, without any thought of it being directly affected by the *NEUROFLOW* from the brain.

We have a circulation system that delivers blood through a network of pipes (arteries and veins), which not only get smaller in diameter but also have acute corners to contend with. The corners are of course, not sharp, they are smoothed out to reduce the angular effect on the flow. Also the blood vessels go against the force of gravity for a great deal of the time.

I would like to compare this setup with something easier for me to understand. An analogy of this could be the pumping of water through a series of flexible pipes, such as a hose used by Fire Brigades. This hose is collapsible, just like blood vessels, and is usually stored in a roll. If several long lengths of such hose were connected together in a single line horizontally and then connected to the outlet of a pump, then water could be pumped to the end of the hose line. This means that the pressure generated by the pump must be enough to overcome the force needed to open up the diameter of the hose, it also has to overcome the frictional loss. The hose would have been flattened due to being in a stored condition and when finally the water reaches the end of the hose line it exits at a pressure. Due to frictional losses and pressure losses due to opening the hose up, the pressure at the end of the line of hose will be less than that at the pump. Now, if further hose lengths are added to the existing line, and a layer of sand is placed on the exterior of the hose lengths and new lines are placed at right angles to the original line, the pressure of the water at the end of the (new, extended and angled) line is even less than that at the pump. We can now add several more new lengths of hose, each reducing in diameter and ending in a diameter which is only 25% of the diameter of the first length of hose that is connected to the pump. Also each section is covered with a layer of sand. We can then raise the end lengths of hose to a vertical position. The pressure reading at the end of the whole line of hose will be negligible. Supposing, the objective of the project was to pump water to a distant place which was also at a high elevation. The purpose might be to turn a water turbine, which requires a water pressure of 80% of that which the pump could produce. The turbine will not work because the pressure loss in the hose line has been too great. Thus the pressure at the turbine may only be 40% of the pump pressure, a loss of 60%, so the turbine does not turn. To make it turn, the pump must turn faster to create greater pressure throughout the system. This raises the available pressure at the turbine to the operating input pressure and it works. The pump however may not be designed to operate like this for long periods and may break, the hose may exceed its designed pressure resistance and burst. Either way the whole system may fail. If a pump produces 10 bar pressure through 30 metres of hose over a level plane and a small nozzle is placed on the end of it, then the water will be expelled through the nozzle. The more lengths of the same hose you add to the line means that the pump has to increase the pressure to overcome a pressure loss in the line (pressure drop) and still maintain the same pressure at the nozzle end, the more lengths of hose added, the worse the problem. If lengths of smaller diameter are added then the pressure drop is even worse. Add corners and rises at the extreme end then the problem is made much worse and eventually water stops flowing. In this case the pressure from the pump is the only thing holding open the hose along its whole length. If we remove the sand however that has been pressing down on the hose, then the pump does not have to work so hard and the pressure in the system is reduced, nothing breaks and the turbine works. This is why firemen take great pains to make calculations when pumping water in awkward situations or over long distances. This is just an example, but does illustrate what I want to say. If we look at the heart and blood circulation system in this way, then something else is removing the 'sand', that is, if blood is to be able to circulate properly. Perhaps the brain has a hand in this. Our whole body is an expression of the brain's activity demands. So in simplified discussion, instruction to and from the brain, which I have already called neuroflow flow, will call these messages up and down through the spinal column and out through the peripheral and autonomic nerves via close association with each vertebra. It then flows through the nervous network to the site of activity, when that activity involves muscles the nerve is called a motor nerve. Where the brain is monitoring the state of the body it needs to receive information about what is required at a particular site. Also it may need to give instruction to another system, an organ system perhaps, to rectify the situation if rectification is required. This is a maintenance procedure. How far does this extend? Does the *NEUROFLOW* extend into the joints or the blood circulation system? It extends throughout the body. No wonder the brain is as big as it is. This sort of thinking is obviously simplified and not looked at through a microscope but on an everyday understandable level, thus it is not in any molecular detail.

Earlier in Chapter 4, I told the story of my arm being injured on the door of a railway carriage. Looking at it again, what happened to my arm from the time of the incident? What was going on? The fact that it hurt was not in doubt. The effect of impact caused damage to the local area on the arm and that fact was transmitted to the brain via the neuroflow flow through the sensory input. The amount of pain felt was proportional to the damage inflicted on the tissue. At the time my immediate reaction was to yell and this ensured that everyone else who was near, knew of my injury. The brain was recognising where the problem was and how bad it was. this fact means that the damage was recognised by the brain. The yell that I gave was the acknowledgement of that fact. My brain therefore knew where the problem was because the eyes had helped to locate it. In addition the pain was being experienced at that exact site and being relayed through the nervous system. Pain is the body's means of telling the client not only where the problem is but also how bad it is. Sometimes this information is supplemented by the eyes. Constant pain means a constantly bad problem and intensity of the pain indicates the severity of the injury.

What had happened to me was that the body had begun its remedial work. Visually, at first, the skin appeared to colour red, which I now know is likely to be the breakage of the local capillaries leaking oxygenated blood. This is what was seen. What was not seen is my theory, which I now lay before you.

Working Theory

For the moment I am carrying on with the event that happened to me as a child. The brain, having accepted the information about the injury to my hand, immediately started to issue instructions via the hypothalamus, which in turn instructed the pituitary gland to begin increasing its production of ACTH (Adrenocorticotrophic Hormone). The sole purpose of ACTH is to instruct the adrenal glands to produce a supply of its normal output of a mixture of materials, including cortisol, glucocorticosteroids, minerolocorticosteriods, androgens and others, all of which I will call ' The Healing Plasma'. In this case, a great deal more healing plasma was produced than usual, because of the emergency situation that existed, and was then secreted into the blood circulation system. The brain closed off the circulation system which did not need the healing plasma in such quantity, to direct the healing plasma to the site of the injury. The healing plasma forms part of the inflammatory process. When it arrived at the site to be repaired it started to coat all the nerves that were in need of attention and the damaged muscles and skin tissue. My brain read the feelings that I experienced through my neural network from my skin sensors. It started to repair and to calm down the damaged nerves so that the brain could regain full monitoring activity. This enabled my brain to bring into play other services from within my body to effect a repair.

This included the ability to carry away the waste products in order to improve the appearance of my arm. Because the monitoring activity of the brain resumed, it then registered the fact that other inflammation in the area of the injury (due to the impact) also needed attention. This situation was read by my brain through the nerves and after a little while, the improved condition of the nerves was relayed back to the brain by the neuroflow. The brain, interpreted the feeling of the repair and expressed it through the senses as 'warmth'. This feeling was not really warmth in terms of conductive heat, but it was clearly the type of feeling that you might get from an exothermic chemical reaction. It felt more like an intense glow and was expressive of the chemical reaction between the healing plasma and the nerves in my arm and hand. This continued for a while then it seemed to cool off. I now believe that the useful power level of the healing plasma was exhausted and so at this point the effect was that the 'heat' started to cool down, this was indicated to the brain as a reduction in warmth at the injury site. When the warmth died down completely the pain level was reduced. This process went on until the repair work being done by the healing plasma was finished and the only reminder of the episode was a large bruise.

This colour change was due to the oxygenated blood being leaked by the damaged blood vessels at the injury site. As it became deoxygenated so the colour of the bruise became a darker red. This was the blood residue. This residue and the damaged tissue was slowly cleared away by the lymphatic clearing system. The old cells (rubbish) were picked up and travelled through the lymphatic system, a collection of tubes. This leads into a lymph node, a place where the lymphatic tube merges with a vein and a membrane is all that separates the blood flow from the lymph. The used cells that were the rubbish collected by the lymphatic system passed through the membrane via the lymph drainage, and into the blood circulation system. This unwanted material was taken round to the liver where it was filtered out, detoxified and deposited into the digestive system. It was then expelled through the digestive tracts. The time element for how long this whole process takes varies according to the severity of the injury, but using my childhood experience as an indicator all the above happened over a period of two days following impact.

This is all very interesting you are probably saying to yourself, but what has all has this got to do with Reflexology? You have very likely had many instances like this where you have injured yourself so perhaps you can relate to what is written here.

Other work I have carried out in my clinic has provided evidence of similar responses to a backache or shoulder pain and various other problems. I therefore suggest that I was experiencing what I call the healing process. In medical terminology this may be known as the inflammatory process. In general, if you hurt yourself, after a while the pain recedes. If the reflex point on the foot hurts when put under treatment pressure, then the problem in the corresponding area in the body gets better. I suggest that we are initiating the same process as described above, the only difference is that in the case of an accident, the response is automatic, whereas in the case of Reflexology it is instructive.

The route via the stimulation of the reflexes on the feet can be thought of in a novel way, in that when the Reflexologist finds that the reflex points on the feet are painful, the brain co- relates this to a specific part of the body. Are we persuading the brain to do something about the problem? I believe we are. From that point, I also believe that a chain reaction is launched. The inflammatory process commences and culminates in the patient feeling warm at the injury site. At first, I found that the proposition that this implies, i.e. that a Reflexologist could be in direct contact with the client's subconscious, rather difficult to comprehend. As time has gone on, I have become more accepting of the fact. Thus where a problem occurs the body recognises it and responds to that problem, the body also clears away the debris and leaves things neat and tidy. This scenario, however, does not always occur, as many patients have an ongoing pain problem that seems to get worse rather than better. In these cases, the body is obviously not responding to the need and maybe this is because the original problem requires time for the body to attend to it, but it does not get that time. It is possible that the pain is worsened by the body doing something which exacerbates the condition. It is also possible that the original injury site has brought on other problems that in turn get worse. The brain cannot see past the original injury site and therefore cannot deal with anything after it, because the neuroflow has been interrupted. There may not therefore be sufficient healing plasma produced by the adrenal glands to deal with the problem completely. Whilst seeing to all the other demands of the body, the amount left to look at the injury site is insufficient. It is this which probably makes the situation worse. The new pain, added to the existing one, creates an even worse pain, the body however might already be in difficulty with the first pain and finds it impossible to eradicate them both. Because the body has to look after the rest of the bodily functions at the same time as attempting to deal with the pain it seems that there is just not enough healing plasma to reduce the pain to zero. The expectation, therefore, may be for long term pain to arise.

An analogy of this is if a bucket is placed under a tap in a kitchen. The normal use of the bucket is to take the water, empty it elsewhere, and then return it to the tap. This keeps the kitchen floor dry. The tap which is in the kitchen, develops a leak because the tap washer needs replacing. Drip by drip the bucket gradually fills, this is seen and the bucket is emptied. Eventually the leak gets worse and the drips get faster. The bucket is not emptied soon enough and the water overflows. A leak appears in the bottom of the bucket and the bucket fills more slowly before it is emptied, it is now not only dripping water onto the kitchen floor but now overflows over the flooring and the damage is done. The tap washer is replaced but the consequences of leaving this have proved to be much greater by ignoring the problem in the first place.

So this maintenance process is going on the whole time inside our bodies, hopefully looking after us throughout our lives, or at least, that is the intention. There seems to be a standard, or blueprint, for the individual. It is against this that the workings of all the individual body's functions are measured. We know that there is a built-in maintenance programme with an automatic built in self-repair system that adheres to that standard. It is not unreasonable to assume that someone must have put it there. It is almost a plan. If so, drawn up by whom? I guess that depends on one's beliefs. The proof of the existence of this blueprint needs further investigation as a concept. Perhaps the answers lie deeper than we as mortals, can hope to reach, but this does not concern me here and is for others to deal with.

Reflexology has its relevance in the healing process by making use of both the stored information in the feet and the normal healing process. During a Reflexology treatment session, usually the client produces a vocal, facial or other movement in response to pain. This is a reaction generated by the pressure applied by the Reflexologist to the client's feet. The client's brain accepts this and co-relates this reflex to the exact position in the body. The pain is a reminder to the brain that the specific area in the body still needs attention. The brain is then persuaded initiate the required reaction. This is the start of the healing process.

The brain starts to close off various arteries, leaving open the route through to the injury site. On arrival, the first job for the healing plasma is to start to repair the nervous system locally and/or at a route along the nerve. This allows the complete passage of neuroflow from the brain to be reinstated thus allowing the healing mechanisms to be carried out.

This healing plasma can be thought of as an ointment that is applied to the nerves. As soon as the healing plasma starts to work the inflammation is reduced. The feedback to the brain through the neuroflow says that the healing process is activated, in use and working. The injury site then starts to feel warm. The initial increase of inflammation is interpreted by the brain as a feeling of warmth (more like a glow) in the area affected. This is a comforting reassurance to the client who is persuaded into thinking, correctly, that something good is happening. After the initial response by the body, the warmth will often 'travel and spread'. For example, a client with a shoulder problem will often feel the warmth not only in the shoulder but also spreading into the neck and down the arm to the elbow and hands. This has to be the healing plasma spreading through the arm via the circulation system.

Sometimes a patient will say that their hands feel warm and yet when the hands are touched, the flesh still feels cold. This is because the nerves are being repaired first. Normal physical heat is not present here and as the injured nerves are repaired the brain is able to see past the original impedance and detect the damage further on. This prompts the brain to issue further instructions to the adrenal glands and more healing plasma is released. The patient can sense this by feeling that the affected area gets warmer or even hotter. The action of the healing plasma on the nerves is what is perceived and reported back to the brain. It is only later that the filament nerves, (also having been coated with the healing plasma) permit the full neuroflow to pass unimpeded. Some of these nerves are connected to the smooth muscle in the wall of the local blood vessels and this stimulates the muscles which are directly attached to the blood vessel walls. As they are excited they stiffen, the blood vessels open up and through the increase in blood flow the flesh starts to feel physically warm. The blood, in larger quantities, carries with it an increased calorific value of body heat. This is discussed more fully in Chapter 8. As the healing plasma gets to the other areas of the site, the muscles, tendons and other tissue parts start to feel the benefit of the healing process. The healing plasma is doing its work well and the client begins to feel better.

In the case where pain is experienced over a period of years, this healing process should have happened a long time ago, but for reasons about which our knowledge is very limited, the body has failed to carry out the necessary work sufficiently. In these cases, the client has progressively accumulated the pain until it becomes bothersome. If nothing is done about it the client fails to acknowledge the difficulty and it continues to worsen. Eventually it may hurt enough to make the client go to the doctor in an attempt to obtain some relief from the pain. By then, the problem may have become acute and structural damage may have occurred. In extreme cases, the problem may have been so bad that no amount of treatment can bring it back to normality. However, if the pain is dealt with effectively and at an early stage and the injury site has been repaired satisfactorily, the prognosis is good. Early indicators to future problems can often be missed. They are giving early warnings and do foretell of trouble ahead, so the need for early attention is paramount. This refers not only to people with back pain, but also to people with many different ailments. These indicators include such things as pain, lumps, heartburn, ulcers, permanently cold hands and feet, stiff backs, and many others.

This is where Reflexology can help by keeping the body in good order and receiving treatment from a professionally trained and adequately qualified Reflexologist. Potential difficulties that may lie ahead can be nipped in the bud.

Under normal circumstances, the adrenal glands can produce about

10mg of cortisol (healing plasma) per day, however, even though they may be called upon to do so, they generally do not produce this amount. Another reason for the failure of the body to carry out its function may be the intervention of clinical drugs. An article appeared in the New Scientist magazine dated November 30th 1996, written by Michael Judge, which I will now paraphrase.

It reported on the hunt for less harmful alternatives to the current anti-inflammatory drugs and their side effects. He was writing in the context of treating the disabling symptoms of Arthritis. This balance of the need to give relief against the side effects is a dilemma for the doctor when they prescribe such drugs as Aspirin and Ibupofen. When pain is felt and a drug is used to relieve it, there is a block created through which the pain cannot travel to the brain for recognition. The patient feels 'better' and assumes that everything is all right. In truth, the cause of the problem is still there, even though it currently causes no pain. This effect may even cause the problem to increase in intensity without the client's awareness. Should another symptom arise at the same site or at another altogether, the natural resulting pain is again masked and the client is unaware. This could be very serious.

An illustration of this was when a woman came to see me for treatment for arthritis in all limbs. During treatment I could get no reaction from her feet and no intercellular pain was felt. I had seen this woman some time before and I knew she should react in the normal way but this was not happening. Even after ten minutes treatment there was still no feeling in her feet, there was no evidence of the healing process in progress. I stopped the treatment and we discussed what had, or rather what had not, happened and I asked her if she had taken any drugs that day. She said that she had taken some Ibuprofen only two hours before seeing me, it was clear that this drug had masked the pain in the body. It also appeared to prevent the chain reaction leading to initiating the healing process. I terminated the session and my client was asked to return the following day when we would try again. The next day, she confirmed that she had taken no drugs at all. Treatment commenced and almost immediately she felt the intercellular pain on the feet in the appropriate areas and three minutes later she could feel the warmth in her limbs. This is clear evidence of the body's own healing mechanism being impeded from carrying out its normal healing process for the benefit of the client.

Perhaps here is a good time to speak a little about the role of endorphins in the management of pain. A person may have had a bad pain but over the years managed to ignore the pain to the point where, to all intents and purposes, the pain drifts away. It may be that a residual stiffness remains but if other pains arise, then they may be dealt with in the same manner. If the normal healing process is unable to deal with the problem(s), then the endorphins, which are the body's own natural pain killers, are brought into play. These appear to mask out the pain element of the injury but leave the damage in place. This is clearly an emergency procedure and not a complete remedy. Repeated treatments of Reflexology can produce new doses of healing plasma for the body to enjoy. Not less than a week should elapse between treatments as this gives the body time to assimilate the treatment and adjust to the new regime. Even in the most acute cases Reflexology stimulates the healing process and makes life a lot more comfortable for the client. After all, a good quality of life is what we all want. So this is how Reflexology works.

Healing Crisis
Considering that Reflexology cannot do any harm to the body because it uses the body's own systems, it seems rather odd that some people go through what we call a healing crisis. This crisis is often quite painful and certainly unwanted. Why does this happen? I have observed many people and talked them through their own experiences. It seems that as we go through life many things happen to a body and we

experience and accumulate pain and discomfort. If the normal healing process cannot deal with the immediate problem it appears that the endorphin activity in the body forms a type of screen and we say that the pain has gone away. In fact, it has not gone away, it is still there, but no pain is felt. Sometimes stiffness will be experienced in the injury site. When a Reflexology treatment is given and the healing system is brought into play the endorphin activity is removed and all the old pains come to the surface, because the healing process is under way and a repair is being affected. After a few days of once again suffering old pains, which appear to be getting worse rather than better, if the client perseveres, the old pains begin to reduce. In this way the old pains are being dealt with at the same time. So when you experience a healing crisis, think it through and you will remember every pain you feel in a chronological order. Such as, "I remember that pain but I thought I had got rid of it a long time ago".

Life-Path Theory

I have wondered about many things during the course of my work as a Reflexologist. There is an abundance of questions about health patterns but it is the answers that are in short supply. In some respects, when working in quite unfamiliar areas of thought, it is possible to believe what you think you know, and yet have a feeling about something that has not yet been identified. The Lifepath Theory raises such feelings. I have talked in the last chapter about maintenance systems and how they look after us during our lives. I have also briefly mentioned the possibility of these systems having to work to a standard. That standard is undoubtedly there in the individual; otherwise all our systems would go haywire. A standard has to be there to serve a purpose, but it is not an end in itself. As an example, a standard for a unit of measurement is necessary so that one person's measurement is the same as another's, thus providing a common equity. Similarly in the body there must be an overall standard to serve the health and wellbeing of an individual and form part of an ideal life. This is how I think of *THE LIFEPATH THEORY*

Following on from previous pages, we now have a proposed answer for the healing process that takes place following a Reflexology treatment. I have seen that clients experience common feelings to each other, note has been taken of the responses of clients in terms of warmth. Now I put forward the Lifepath Theory that requires a standard to which all the body's organs must perform. In order to do this the maintenance systems must work and then stop working to the value of that standard, to bring the person back to the Lifepath.

In every sense, the Lifepath is essential for a healthy life and if we keep to this course then nothing will intervene to remove us from it. All our internal systems for maintenance must be working perfectly to achieve a standard which is built into the brain, this standard is the way to follow the Lifepath. I have come across people who seem to have sailed through life without any apparent health difficulties at all. One woman comes to mind who came to me supposedly for treatment, but who in fact she just loved having her feet massaged. There were no prominent reflexes on either foot. She confirmed that she had given birth to two children, both of whom were born within two hours of labour. Her menstruation cycle had been 'perfect'. A happy marriage, up to this point, and a reasonable standard of living had given this person a very happy life. She had absolutely no worries at all. Similarly, I can think of at least one man who just wanted to 'try' Reflexology, he had no prominent reflexes, he was very happy with his life and health, although his financial situation was sometimes a minor cause of stress. In both cases they had been lucky in that they had been able to follow the Lifepath without hindrance.

It is not given for all of us to be so fortunate. In fact most of us get some illness or other during our lives, and if we do, then this is where our maintenance systems carry out their work to put us back on the Lifepath. Unfortunately, this does not always happen. Some of us will contract arthritis, osteoporosis, heart disease, cancer or other chronic disease. The big question is why? I cannot prescribe a panacea for all evils, but for a number of 'internal' diseases there may be another way of looking at them. The Lifepath is present in all of us. Without it there is no purpose for the standard that provides the parameters for the maintenance systems.

Over many Reflexology treatment sessions I have begun to develop new areas for the Reflexology reflex and this has speeded up the whole recovery process. I have noted a relationship between the rate of recovery and the intensity of the warmth that is part of the inflammatory process. This is not a rigid pattern but most people fit into this category. A general guide to the intensity of the warmth has been noted. In children and teenagers and people in their early twenties, mostly seemed to report very intense heat. People in their late twenties to late forties seemed to report a medium to less intense heat. After the age of approximately fifty the heat value is still strong but decreases a little with age. The severity of the problem, no matter at what age, will produce an intensity of heat commensurate with the damage. There are always exceptions to the rule and there have been people in their seventies and some older, who have experienced very intense heat. Why this should be so needs very great research.

Undoubtedly the adrenal glands look after our physical wellbeing throughout our lives. The two things in our lives that are absolutely certain are that we were born and we will die. Therefore the Lifepath has a finite timespan. As we grow from birth our body adapts and heads towards maturity and we are aware that we reach a peak of life's maturity at a certain age, usually in the twenties. There is an uncompromising decline as we go on into old age, when the body systems do not work as well as they used to. The repair systems slow down until everything stops at death. It is logical then, that as we journey on to life's end our physical activity decreases and so does the ability of the adrenal glands' maintenance systems. However, even at the later stage of life the power to repair is still present albeit at a reduced level. I have treated people in their eighties and nineties and still they feel the warmth after a Reflexology treatment.

So what are these systems, the maintenance systems that some call the defence mechanisms, that keep us on the Lifepath?

They are -
1. The Immune System - to fight invading viruses;
2. The Inflammation System - the healing process system - to fight inflammation;
3. The Evacuation System - kidney and liver-digestive systems;
4. The Lymphatic System - to wash, bathe and drain all tissue, to collect all debris generated in the body and deposit it into the blood circulation system;
5. The Blood Circulation System - to carry oxygen, nutrients, products of the immune and healing systems to all parts of the body deposited in it by the lymphatic system.
6. The Nervous System - this is the means by which the brain controls all aspects of the body's physical functions. The nerves carry instructive information, (neuroflow), receive and transmit back to the brain all sensory information. Generally this is loosely described as 'Bio-feedback', but this description tends to isolate a specific function, whereas the feedback aspect is only part of the overall function of the distribution of all information.

Although these systems can be described as individual, in fact they all work as a team. Not only that, they always have to work in combination with each other in response to the needs of the body to get back to the Lifepath. All this is co-ordinated by the brain, which uses the Lifepath as the goal. When I look at the above I realise that the whole body is working in concert and is interdependent on itself as a whole.

Reflexology looks at the body in much the same way and we call it 'Holistic', that is, treating the whole body and not just part of it. This is a statement which doctors find difficult to accept. If you have a pain in the big toe of a foot the doctor will tend to treat the symptoms surrounding the toe by blocking the pain with analgesics. Speaking as a Reflexologist, treatment should start with the whole of the skeletal system before attending to the rest of the body on the feet, then pains on the feet (reflexes) would undoubtedly become apparent. These would relate to the problem in the body that may reflect the root of the difficulty of which the client is complaining. The Lifepath demands that there should be no problem with the body and consequently neither with the big toe and so the brain brings in the inflammatory process which initiates the healing process and the pain goes away because the inflammation in the body is eliminated. As this happens the intercellular pain in the big toe also reduces. Thus the body as a whole is brought back to the Lifepath and health and wellbeing are re-established.

The problem now is what happens to the majority of us who have had previous accidents or menstrual difficulties? Let me illustrate what can happen when I recall the case of a particular woman who came to me for help. She had experienced a difficult time with her menstrual cycle ever since her periods began. This fact had taken her away from the Lifepath and because nothing could be done to rectify the problem, she stayed away from it. She had had a car accident and suffered whiplash in her neck. The menstrual problem was still with her. Later she started to get feelings of panic that nobody could explain. Some years after the accident the neck problem had worsened and had started to give her pain in the right shoulder. Her right elbow was now hurting and she was having pain in her right hand. When she came to me she was feeling very low.

What was happening was that from an early age she was straying from the Lifepath. The body could not deal with the situation at that time so it got on with the maintenance of the rest of her body. When the car accident occurred the whiplash caused damage to the brachial group of nerves which go from the cervical vertebrae in the neck down the arms, terminating in the tips of the fingers. In addition the whiplash damaged the whole of the nerve network in the shoulder which was now giving her pain. Again, she had already moved away from the Lifepath and now there was an additional problem that took her even further away. Her body's defences tried to deal with the problem but were unable to cope. Once more she was now even further away from the Lifepath and the problems stayed with her. Instead of staying the same, when the situation was not corrected the problem worsened, hence the pains in her elbow and hand. When giving her repeated Reflexology treatments she was able to feel the warmth intensely in her neck and shoulder and the rest of the arm. Week by week she was able to report a gradual improvement in the shoulder until she had no pain at all. Her menstrual cycle had also become 'normal'. Warmth had also been reported in her lower back and tummy. Throughout the treatment sessions the warmth in these areas also reduced. Clearly there had been a problem in her lower back for years (she agreed with this) but she had ignored it this meant that the normal connection from the brain down to the uterus and ovaries had been interrupted by the inflammation in the lower back. The neuroflow pattern was incomplete and the brain could not see that there was a problem; therefore, there could be no comparison with the standard. By using Reflexology I had removed the impedance by removing the inflammation. This allowed the brain at last to see what was wrong and it brought in all the necessary systems to correct things. The ovaries and uterus were put into a much better condition and the client felt the benefit. By returning to the Lifepath she had become more active and felt more alive. This was because the body was now functioning normally and complied with the standard demanded by the Lifepath.

Another woman came to me and said that she had been medically diagnosed with osteoarthritis in the hips and knees. It had started with a very painful lower back for which she had been to her doctor who had prescribed rest and painkillers. This had had a marginal effect on her pain, so more powerful painkillers were prescribed. These worked a little better for a while but their effectiveness, as far as pain reduction was concerned, was diminishing. She was prescribed a total of twelve weeks physiotherapy, at the end of which some relief was experienced, but the pain soon returned. By this time this woman was getting cramp in both legs and her feet were very cold. She was referred to a pain clinic where she was offered more pain killers and then an epidural injection. By now her knees were beginning to hurt greatly and her mobility was also curtailed. She came to me to see if I could help with pain. By this time she had been diagnosed as being arthritic and had been offered replacement knees and hips, but she would have to wait for this to be done. She had X-rays taken to see what was going on, but the osteoarthritis was not so bad. Does any of this sound familiar?

The woman came to me and I applied a full treatment to both feet, but went back to reinforce the treatment on the spine, and lower back reflexes, with determination. After about twenty minutes her lower back began to warm up, as did her legs and hips. After some forty minutes, the intensity of the heat was reducing. When she was about to leave she reported that her pain level was reduced and she was still warm. Subsequent visits reduced the pain even further until she could walk into and around town, and then home again. She could pick up her grandchild more easily and overall her quality of life had improved a great deal.

The progression of deterioration can be seen in this example. Ache in the lower back becomes worse over the years, meanwhile her hips hurt and her feet are always cold. She gets cramp and her knees hurt.

If we look at this in reverse, we have the knees, cramp, hips and lower back. There is progressive activity here. Supposing we could stop the ache in the lower back, then probably we could stop the hips and knees hurting and getting worse, and we could also prevent the cramp. From little acorns do big oak trees grow.

To understand this a little better, try to imagine an old clock. This relies on a tensioned spring and a series of cogs with teeth that interconnect and ultimately turn a spindle which rotates the hands around the clock face. I am leaving out all sorts of things but the example is best seen in simplistic terms. When the spring is wound up with a key, the stored energy turns the cogs at the correct speed. All the teeth are carefully arranged so that all movement is smooth with each cog playing its part in the process. If a cog is incorrectly machined its teeth will 'chatter' against its neighbour. This makes no difference to the running of the clock in the short term but as the clock ages the chatter is increased and the next cog creates chatter, and so on. What started as a small problem has grown into a major problem. The clock goes wrong and a trip to the horologist is necessary. During its life the clock has always told the time but with increasing unreliability.

This could be seen to be representing the pattern of our lives. Damage or small injuries which occur frequently in early life and appear as unimportant to us at the time, can all too often grow into something much bigger in later life. So that the concept of the Lifepath can be more easily identified I would like to relay the case of a man who came to see me.

I was outside my house when this person caught my attention and we had the consultation in my driveway. He told me that he was unwell, that he had been to his doctor with symptoms that caused his GP to send him to hospital. He was given an M.R.I scan that revealed an enlargement of his liver, there was nothing that could be offered to him for treatment except to keep in touch with his doctor. Another appointment with the hospital was made and he was sent home. He asked me if there was anything that I could do. This was the 'last chance saloon', he did not know what was possible but was now in a position where any help would be welcome I wanted to help if it was at all possible and so I asked him if he was prepared to listen to my theories and how they may be applied to him, he agreed. We went to my treatment room and I began the consultation by telling him that in my opinion there was a reason for everything. His case was no different to any other in that respect, we just had to find the reason for his problem. I asked how long ago it was that he first felt unwell and when he had received the diagnosis. He said that he first felt poorly about seven months ago, the hospital diagnosis was two months after that. I asked him if he had experienced any pain in the cervical or upper and central thoracic sections of the spine and he confirmed this was so. He told me that he had suffered much in the way of pain in what turned out to be the central thoracic spine area and his neck. The pain was so bad that he had visited the doctor on several occasions about it but had not been able to do anything to reduce the pain level, in the end the pain did subside a little, naturally. I asked how he had got the pain in the first place and he told me that he had been in the attic of his house and he had fallen from the opening. Whilst falling feet first, he managed to save himself by holding on to the side of the attic opening with both hands. As he came to a halt, the pull of gravity and his weight, stretched his back and arms. It was about two weeks after this that he began to feel the pain in his upper and central back. As the pain grew in intensity it started to spread from the spine to come around to his sides.

I explained that in my opinion, the fall that happened had stretched his spine and had badly disturbed the stream of neuroflow through the system of nerves. These nerves get smaller and smaller, ending with the filament nerves that are normally connected to the liver. The Lifepath dictated that the liver was to function perfectly with no difficulty. To do this, the standard set the parameters within which a person could live without knowledge of what was going on and therefore live a normal life. The parameters for the liver would be such as what colour it should be and what size it should be, the condition of the liver was most important because it determined how it carried out its functions. In his case the neuroflow had been impeded at the spine and at the autonomic system in the area. The liver was not receiving enough neuroflow and so it did its own thing and as there was no correction and the standard could not be enforced, it enlarged. It still carried out its function as a liver, albeit with diminishing ability, but the lack of neuroflow allowed the liver to increase in size.

Not unexpectedly, my patient was a little sceptical about my explanation. He had not come across this way of thinking before, however, he asked me to carry out treatment. We commenced that week and I applied treatment to the reflexes corresponding to the pituitary and the whole spine, with particular emphasis on the cervical and thoracic sections, the shoulders and the arms. We waited for the healing plasma to arrive at the site of the upper back. Within two minutes his spine T1-T5 and C5-C7 started to feel warm. Five minutes later he said the warmth was now hot. His shoulder and neck was also feeling hot and his arms were warm. About ten minutes later he could feel warmth coming around the sides of his chest and this continued for another five minutes when he said something that surprised me. He said he could feel warmth inside his upper chest, above the waist. He could feel the warmth spreading inside his trunk and he could feel the outline of the liver inside the body. We were both looking at each other with amazement. He said that he felt no discomfort; in fact it was a most comforting feeling. This went on for about twenty minutes. The 'hot' feeling reduced in stages to a pleasant, cosy feeling. At the end of the session he was back to normal in terms of heat. We discussed what had happened and he was beginning to see that I might be right in my assessment and treatment.

I treated him in exactly the same way for another three weeks. By this time the warmth was reducing steadily and no more could be felt in his upper back and liver on the fourth week. I was expecting him to arrive as arranged on the fifth week but he did not show up, in fact I did not see him for three months and then to my delight, I saw him in the street in my town. We said our hellos and he said that he had broken his leg and had been out of action for three months. I asked about the liver and his hospital visit. He said that the hospital had done a new M.R.I scan. They could not understand it because it showed that the liver (which had been described by them as being huge) had returned to normal size. The hospital staff said that it must have done this by itself and passed it off. He had told them that it was due to the treatment I had given to him, but there was no further comment. My patient was clearly overjoyed and I was very pleased as well. In a way, the liver had responded quite naturally with a little help from me, no drugs or surgery had been necessary. The healing process had repaired the neural network at the injury site and the brain had regained full control of the situation. It realised that something was wrong and quickly brought into play more of the healing processes to care for the liver and provide the parameters to which the liver should comply and this brought it back to its normal size. This was imposing the standard on the liver so that my patient could again restore himself to the Lifepath.

Another case illustrates this very well. A woman came to me for treatment for a long-standing pain in her lower back. Using my method of the application of Reflexology, which I call NEUROFLEXOLOGY, the usual results of heat and warmth were experienced by her until on a particular day in September 1997 she told me that she had to visit a hospital about a prolapsed rectum and she was very upset about the recommendation for surgery. I explained in brief, my theory and she jumped at the chance of natural recovery. I worked on her weekly for thirteen weeks. Each treatment successfully brought about a feeling of heat that started in the lumbar/sacrum areas of the spine and gradually spread across her lower back. I realised what was going to happen and we both waited for the process to progress and it did. At first the lower back stayed warm, then the warmth began to intensify all over the lower back. She then found that the heat was spreading from her lower back, to inside her abdominal cavity. Her buttocks got warm and she could feel the warmth moving inside her vagina and rectum. This warmth stayed with the patient for thirty-five minutes, then it started to reduce in temperature and stopped at a comfortable level. She left after some forty-five minutes, still warm. The following week, she reported that there was no appreciable change in her discomfort, but her lower back was very much better. Again treatment was given and again the same heat was generated in the abdomen, the vagina and rectum. The following week the same thing happened, but this time she said she could feel something moving in her abdomen. Her comfort level had improved. For some eight weeks, this same process went on and her comfort level was improving all the time. By the eleventh week, she came into my treatment room and was very pleased to tell me that not only was her back very well, but her comfort level was 98% normal. She was delighted and said that clearly my theory was proving correct. The twelfth week arrived and with the same treatment applied it produced only slight warmth in the whole abdomen and pelvic floor and she confirmed that now she felt no discomfort at all. The following week, she had no discomfort and no heat and since then she has seen me and confirmed that everything was now normal.

Clearly in this case, her long-standing lower back condition had been building up the inflammation around the lumbar and sacrum areas. This in turn engulfed the autonomic system in that area. It had part blocked the neuroflow and the brain could not see past the inflammation. This prevented the brain from seeing and remedying what had gone wrong in whole or in part. The filament nerves from the ganglia are attached to the spinal vertebra. They form part of the autonomic system and had been damaged over many years due to the lack of maintenance. The brain was not calling on the adrenal glands to send the healing plasma down to the area identified by the filament nerves. This area might be the muscle structure and intestines or, in this case, the rectum. The geographical position of the rectum was eventually lost. That portion of the intestine parted from the surrounding connective tissue and the vaginal canal had also weakened; the result was a prolapsed rectum that was allowed to flop over. With weekly treatments the neural system began to reconnect to the rectum. As it did so gradually the rectum began to return to where it came from. It had been repaired up to the point of normality.

I have treated other women who have had, in addition to other problems, prolapsed wombs. All the other problems seemed to clear up nicely, but the impact on the prolapsed womb was not positive. In each case, the prolapse had existed for a long time before the client came to see me. There is clearly a relationship between the length of time that a prolapse first occurs and the effectiveness of this treatment. The longer a prolapse has been in existence the less likely the body can effect a repair as explained in the above case. However, if caught in the early stages there is no doubt in my mind that a similar outcome to that above could be expected. The blueprint in our brains, that I call the standard, can bring the client back to normality for the age of that client and can return the client to the Lifepath for a healthier life. In the above case, the woman's brain knew that the prolapse was wrong when compared with the standard and because the conditions were still in place to restore the rectum to its proper place, a repair was possible. The client had benefited and comfort was the result. The Lifepath is the ultimate and most ideal way through life that the body can achieve. The working theory is the means by which this can be achieved.

To illustrate this even further, I would like to highlight the case of a man who had played rugby as a youngster and had injured his back during one match. He had recovered somewhat, but his back still gave him trouble. He went to various therapists and was told that his hips had moved out of alignment and this had affected his spine and shoulder alignment. Treatment had been given and to a large extent the pain had reduced. The man was learning to live with it and until recently he had learned to cope reasonably well. He was a man who had had a successful life as a director of one or more companies. He confessed that he had no idea of what he was about to embark upon. The injury occurred when he was fourteen years and he was now seventy-six years of age. This had left him with his shoulders inclining down to the left and his hips inclining down to the right, but in spite of this affliction he had been able to lead a successful life in business. He said that he had suffered with very bad headaches and neck pain for years and these pains were getting worse. Over a period of years he had received treatment from a chiropractor which had helped him a lot in easing the pain in his neck, but only for a very short time, usually a day, sometimes longer. His daughter had told him to see a Reflexologist and he decided to come to see me.

Listening to him talk I formed a picture in my mind about what had happened during the intervening years. Clearly, with the hips being angled, his lower back would have been painful, which would also explain the neck and head pains. As he had not been born like this and as my knowledge of the Lifepath theory was present in my mind, I told the man that we may be able to restore the hips and shoulders to being level, which would relieve the pain in his lower back and shoulders; although I also told him that there was no guarantee but things did look hopeful. It was for him to decide to go on or not. He agreed that we start straight away.

The treatment lasted over a period of months and although too involved to relate here, I will describe some of the events that took place.

Initially, this patient experienced, as in all other cases, the feeling of warmth in his whole spine but particularly around his neck and sacro iliac joint. Clearly, these were the two major junctions that had been badly affected by his accident all those years before. Heat was also present in his neck and back of his head. As time went by his neck began to ease slightly but not totally. He told me that he knew that only when his shoulders were level and the repair work was completed would his neck be free of pain. On one occasion he came to my clinic and told me that whilst out walking one day he felt that his whole trunk was being forced to twist to the left. He realised that something major was happening to him, and so did I.

We continued for a few more weeks and he again reported that he had experienced his head being twisted around to the right. This could only mean that with all of the repair work that had been going on his body was able to refer to the standard. His brain was now checking that it could see what was going on with the newly repaired nerves. Realising that everything was out of place, it gave instructions for the muscles to physically pull his body back into shape when compared with the blueprint for his body. It was doing something major to return it to the standard's fixed parameters. In other words, his body was being put back to where it should be, had it not been for that accident years before. The Lifepath was beginning to be attainable. What is more, his shoulders and hips have remained level ever since. This is a graphic case of a body being adjusted back to where it should have been. The standard had been used as a yardstick in order to return him to a more comfortable life.

Rethinking Reflexology   by   John C F Moorhouse

Chapter 6

Proof

The proof of the pudding is in the eating. Some pudding! It can often be seen in books on Reflexology cases where, following treatment, this or that client got better. All of which may be real to the Reflexologist and the client, but it is only treated as anecdotal by the medical profession. Currently, much more notice is being taken of such evidence due to the sheer weight of it. However, apart from trials where a large number of people are involved, we can put forward cases where hospitals or individual physicians confirm that an event has taken place. Even in large trials where control and placebo groups are used, these are now being questioned. So where does this leave us? Perhaps something would turn up and help me prove one or more of my theories. Well, something did, and this was what I had waited for.

I had a phone call from a woman who was calling on behalf of her husband, George. She said she had been recommended by her friend to contact me. Poor George, he had such a terrible problem with his back that he could hardly move. She did not know quite how she was going to get him over to me as the car ride would hurt him a great deal. Anyway she made the appointment and I waited for them to arrive. They both turned up and I could see George passing my window very, very slowly. He eventually came into my treatment room and I could see the agony on his face. Every move he made resulted in agonising pain. His wife was clearly worried. I invited George to sit in my treatment chair , which although initially he said he couldn't, he did manage with some courage. The design of the chair meant that all his weight was held and no effort to support his body was necessary. He told me that he had been to see a consultant and specialist and an X-ray had been taken, the results of which he had brought with him.

I could see clearly that he had a prolapsed intervertebral disc (a slipped disc). His wife asked what I could do for him. I explained my theories and advised them that treatment was worth pursuing. They agreed.

I concentrated the treatment on his feet, around the spine and new areas that I have discovered for the sciatic nerves. We waited for a few minutes and he started to feel warmth in his lower back. The intensity of heat grew until it seemed to him to be overwhelming his pain. After a few minutes more he felt warmth filling his abdomen and travelling down each leg. This process carried on until it started to 'cool down'. This was about twenty-five minutes later. By the time forty-five minutes had elapsed he could feel a lesser but very comfortable warmth from his waist down to his feet. At this point he expressed a little more comfort in his back and he sat more easily in the chair. We began to talk and George looked incredulously at me and asked what I had done to him to produce that result. I explained my working theory again and although he did not fully understand all of it, he accepted my explanation. George and his wife left my treatment room, having first made another appointment for the following week. George seemed to be moving with less trouble than when he arrived. I saw him pass the window again and this time he was walking in a much improved manner.

The following week, George and his wife returned. I had arranged extra time for him because I guessed there would be a lot to talk about and I was right. George walked into my treatment room without hanging onto the wall. He sat down with care but with more ease than the previous week. He smiled at me and started to tell me what had happened over the previous seven days. He had gone home in the car with his wife driving and he still felt warmth in his back. The amount of pain he was suffering had reduced, but he still hurt at a lower level. He then began to tell me his history. He started to feel a great deal of pain in his back and he went to his doctor. His doctor examined him and he was referred to a consultant at a well-known hospital. The first letter was dated 26th September 1996 and was followed by another letter shortly after. This was followed by an analysis of DTS-referral. After this, George began to deteriorate fast and a good friend recommended him to come and see me. The treatment commenced on the 5th February 1997.

By the third treatment, his pain level had been lowered and he was beginning to rethink his future. Before we started treatment, he told me that he had planned a holiday in the USA and thought about buying a house in France. Up to then he was looking at wheelchairs for the rest of his life, but now he was much more positive about recovery and was booking the holiday and going over to France later to look at a house to purchase. None of these tasks would have been possible or in such a quick time before the treatment. The progression of letters between the two doctors handling George's case was significant in their content. The diagnosis they had arrived at was heading for surgical intervention. The later letter shows confirmation of recovery. The final letter is written again by a doctor whom George had attended for plain X-ray films of his thoraco-lumber junction. The doctor was able to chat to him that afternoon. The doctor's letter read;

"The patient really does appear to be in very good health, with minimal residual discomforts. Coned views of the D12/L1 region were performed. This shows a slight increase in bone density at the ill defined intervertebral disc space. Further development of anterior osteophytic beaking. There is no additional adverse feature to suggest reactivation of sepsis. The rest of his visualised thoraco-lumber spine shows some moderate degenerative change only. CONCLUSIONS. Slight but definite further progression of boney healing. I took the liberty to show George his films this afternoon. I hope this helps you in the your continued clinical management".
Kind regards.

This is proof of the effects of my treatment of George between 16th January 1997 and 12th June 1997. George had taken no drug therapy or any other form of therapy except coming to me for Reflexology treatment. I would say that this is - PROOF POSITIVE.

Out of courtesy, I wrote to the consultant and sent a copy of what I had written in this book about George. He eventually replied and said that he would not be very happy with what I had written. He said that experts had predicted a spontaneous resolution to George's problem. However, George had previously told me that a doctor had told him that it was not possible for the body to recover so quickly. In this case, the body was helped to make a rapid recovery by the Reflexology treatment it had received. This cannot be ignored.

Another example can be found in Arthur. Arthur is a sixty-nine year old man who had suffered with his heart for forty years. It had ruled his and his family's lives. He was unable to walk more than two hundred paces before he became very tired and breathless, and he was unable to carry out the most simple of tasks without discomfort. All the help he would love to have given to his children and wife could not be given and it had become a source of acute frustration to him.

Arthur heard me on a local radio show, during which I said that I had a theory about how people get heart attacks. I asked for anyone listening to call me. Many did. One man phoned me and said that he had been checking with thirteen members of his family. He told me that without exception, all thirteen had heart problems and angina, so it obviously ran in the family. The common link with the people who phoned me was that they all suffered with arthritis in the neck (spondylosis) and some with pain in the left shoulder. Arthur spoke to me at length and said he wanted to try out my theories to see if I could do what conventional medicine had failed to do.

We commenced treatment for his aches and pains, including the pain in his cervical spine (neck) and left shoulder. He was currently taking six different types of drug for the control of his heart/angina condition, and was being monitored about every two years by a hospital. One such visit was due five weeks following his first visit to me. He experienced the heat (healing plasma, as described previously), in his neck and left shoulder and on his chest. This was clearly the healing plasma getting at the spondylosis in his neck, thus allowing the brain to see past the inflammation. The route from the spine along the autonomic system, via the filament nerves, leading to the heart, was then opened. The brain could see that the heart needed attention. The healing plasma was sent further along the nerves to the heart. This accounted for the warm feeling the patient felt on his chest. He felt an even warmer position in his chest, where his heart was located. The blood supply carrying the healing plasma to the blood system for the heart and the plasma was distributed over the surface of the heart. In this respect, the method used by the body to carry out repairs was no different to the repair of any other organ.

This process of treatment was carried out in the same manner for three weeks. On his fourth visit, he told me that he had been able to mend his daughter's fridge. He was able to clear her lawn of leaves, and to walk around Coventry and do the shopping. All this was done without any ill affects and without becoming unduly breathless. He was clearly elated. The following week he was due to visit the hospital and he went as arranged. The staff were a little surprised at his ability to perform so well on the apparatus. They told him that the read-out showed that there was no evidence of the angina, or of any heart irregularity. The next three weeks saw the heat in the neck reduced until there was none. The patient was very happy. This is a clear case supporting everything said before in this book and confirms that angina and many heart problems can be dealt with naturally without recourse to surgery or drug therapy. This is a clear case of the body returning to the Lifepath, by repairing the nerve connection between the heart and the brain and restoring the heart to its operational condition. The proof of this came after Arthur was asked to visit a consultant who had attended his case for some time. Arthur was asked to have a CT scan and a X-ray for his condition. He did and the consultant told him that he was surprised but pleased to tell him that he *no longer had angina, nor were his arteries blocked.* Arthur was over the moon with delight and he could not wait to tell me. He said that if he had not listened to me on the radio on that day, listened to my theories and come to see me, he might never have recovered his health.

What good are theories if they do not profit the client?

Of course not all people with heart conditions will have these symptoms, but this example may well apply to very many people. Even those who say that they have no problem in their neck, in my experience, may still have the same symptoms, even though they do not acknowledge them. The feet, however, tell a different tale.

Chapter 7

Leg and Arm
Arthritis

There are about 200 varieties of arthritis but we cannot deal with them all here. If a client comes to see me and says that he or she has rheumatoid arthritis in the left shoulder and arm, the type of arthritis is not important to me in this context. We classify the type of arthritis as people, but it is irrelevant to the brain and the fact that a client has a pain in the shoulder and arm is enough. It is we who give names to various classes of arthritis. The parts of the brain that operate the maintenance systems in the body have no such classification. Armed with what I have written here and the experience I have gained from my work as a Reflexologist, I know that the body can help itself with an internal problem, whatever it is called. I now want to explore the following problems as reported by my clients.

By far most of the clients I see visit the clinic as a result of pains in the legs and lower back - backache and twinges in the lower back (lumbar and sacrum areas) and pain across the lower buttock. We can add to these areas, although sometimes they appear separately - hip pain, pain in the side around the waistline, pains or aching in the thighs, painful knees, numb places on the legs or toes, jumpy legs, cramp and others. This is quite a list to us, but not to the brain as it sees them only as part of the same problem. Swelling of the legs and/or ankles is often evident. We can add to the list stiff, painful or frozen shoulders, painful elbows, painful wrists, hands and fingers that hurt etc. The swelling of the knuckles, elbows and hands may also accompany any of the above. Also a more common complaint which I encounter is osteoarthritis. Occasionally some patients complain of pain in the actual joints and have assumed that they have 'arthritis', but the client has never bothered to obtain a doctor's diagnosis. These people I always advise to see their doctor before I carry out any treatment. Accompanying these symptoms there is usually coldness in the hands and feet, and there is a real link with all of these symptoms.

Legs and lower back - Arthritis

Normally, if we have arthritic backache or our knees hurt, on visiting a surgery the doctor will centre their attention around the knee or back problems individually. Indeed, this is the procedure adopted by hospital departments. When you look at this a pattern begins to emerge. A client will often complain to me about knees hurting and totally ignore the fact that their lower back is very painful or stiff. Once people get into pain, as previously indicated, a long road of medication lies ahead. In my experience, most people expect pain in their 'old age' - THIS NEED NOT NECESSARILY BE THE CASE! There is no need to dread an old age that is associated with pain. Comfort is possible. Bearing in mind that the brain controls and monitors every function in the legs and lower back. The whole of the leg structure and to much extent the lower back is functioning continuously like a live wire, receiving information and giving instruction (neuroflow). Therefore muscles have no intelligence. If they did, for example, after the nerve structure has been withdrawn from a leg the muscles would still function. They plainly do not. The muscles then need to be told what to do. These instructions are continually being issued by the brain to feed instructions to the muscles. How does it do this? The brain's only direct connection with the legs is down the spinal column, out through the lumbar and sacrum and along what is called, the sciatic group of nerves. Neuroflow also travels through the whole of the nerve system.

In the legs, the sciatic nerves meet the spine at the sacrum and lumbar sections, a very busy junction. In the case of the arms, the brachial nerves exit the spine at the cervical section (the neck area). We tend to call the area where the sciatic nerves and the spine is located, the lower back. Most often it is this area that aches. If muscles misbehave, as with cramp, it is because the neuroflow is not getting the messages through to the brain in their entirety. Because the muscles are not given clear and precise information they revert back to their prearranged state of rigidity and the pain is a warning for us to do something about it; i.e. relieve the impedance on the sciatic nerves. The stream of neuroflow may be hindered by obstructions on the nerves. This impedance could be inflammation or pinching of the nerve anywhere in its length up to the muscle. When a client experiences cramp, it is highly likely that they have had a lower backache or stiffness in the lower back for some considerable time. Here I am excluding the effects of accidental damage, although even here the principle is the same.

This possibility of the interference of the neuroflow causing a malfunction further down the line may have extensive ramifications. This whole idea of the brain monitoring and controlling functions in the legs is graphically illustrated by the case of a woman called Iris. She was training to become a Reflexologist and she had heard me talk about my theories. Iris told me that an accident in 1979 had left her with a very painful lower back with right sided sciatic pain. In 1983 she had an event in her life that resulted in her experiencing numbness of the right foot. She was in such pain that she went to see her doctor who referred her to a local hospital. There a consultant orthopaedic surgeon saw her. He wrote a letter to a consultant neurosurgeon at a Centre for Neurosurgery & Neurology in England, dated 1st October 1985 and the letter is reproduced here. Note the reference to the wasting of the right calf.

"I would be obliged if you would see this patient who developed lower back pain and acute right sided sciatica in October 1984. The pain appeared to clear up by December but she continued to

have progressive weakness in her right leg and numbness in the leg and foot. She now only has a moderate amount of low back pain and persistent weakness in her leg. Her straight leg raining is 90° on both sides. There is significant wasting in her right calf with numbness in the SI dermatome. The right ankle jerk is absent.

I had E.M.G. studies carried out and I enclose a copy of the results. She recently had a radiculogram, which showed no disc prolapse at the L5/SI level but a small central disc prolapse at the L4/5 level. The question remains as to whether the weakness in the right lower limb is due to permanent root lesion or whether something further can be done to alleviate her symptoms.

I would appreciate your help and advice on the matter. I enclose her myelogram as well.

Yours sincerely. "

Tests were conducted on Iris. In reply to the letter from the consultant orthopaedic surgeon, the consultant neurosurgeon wrote his reply dated 15th November 1985, which is quoted below. It will be noted that an operation was not advised.

"Thank you for your letter about this patient. I gather her history of back trouble goes back for about 4 years, with recurring episodes of low back pain and right sided sciatica and with numbness of the right foot persisting since a particularly severe event in 1983. At the present time she still complains of this sciatic pain but it is accompanied by severe evidence of right first sacral root with absent ankle jerk and both motor and sensory impairment. The myelogram does not show any gross lesion at this level, though the disc space is markedly collapsed. She does have a markedly wide dura at the L5/SI level so I think while she

must have had an extruded disc fragment, this is probably now flattened and adherent and I rather fear that exploration might well do more harm that good at this stage.The disc space is so collapsed that I think it unlikely that she will have any further material to extrude. In these circumstances I would not advise operation at this stage."

Iris was still left with the pain and other symptoms mentioned in the letter above. Her doctor told her that she should learn to live with it as there was nothing more that could be done and an operation was not advisable. Iris then went on with the rest of her life. Her condition worsened until her right heel became very painful and was without any actual feeling. She was losing almost all feeling in the whole of her right leg and the wasting of her calf muscle continued. Despite the far reaching problem that was presented to me, the thing which she complained of most, was her painful heel. She described the heel as feeling as if it had a solid steel core, and it was extremely cold.

So it was when Iris came to see me she was walking with a slight limp on the right side. I feel that I should say here that it was not the fault of her doctors that nothing was done. Within the limits of their training they did all that could be expected. Going back over the historical progression of her difficulties it was clear that the sciatic nerves were in trouble. I told Iris that no guarantee could be given but I felt that there was a good chance that at least some relief would be experienced.

We started treatment and waited for her body to respond. The sciatic reflexes on both feet were very painful and the spinal reflexes for the lumbar, sacral and coccyx sections were painful on the right foot only. About four minutes later she began to feel warmth in her lower back. Iris was very aware of her body and had no difficulty in identifying what was happening inside her body relating to the 'heat' and tingling.

Iris told me that she could feel heat going across her back and then across part of the inside of her right buttock. She could also identify tingling from her sacrum to her right hip, and then the tingling would travel down the underneath of her right thigh. Her knee tingled a great deal and her thigh was a little warm. This process would carry on and at one time her right heel was tingling. At this point she was almost in tears. I think that this was because she had believed that nothing could be done about her heel, yet it was tingling. We finished the session and she was close to tears, but very happy.

The next session started and she began to warm up in the lower back quicker than before, after only three minutes. The 'heat' continued across her back and into her right buttock. It then travelled into her right thigh and then her right knee warmed up. While all this was going on, she told me that if she touched the back of her thigh it felt as though her hand was about twelve inches away from her thigh. She was giving me regular reports on the progress of the 'heat' and the tingling. By now it had reached her right foot but the right heel was unaffected. Several other treatments followed in the ensuing weeks and all the time the depth and quality of 'heat' increased. Progress was made towards the 'recovery' of the right leg and tangible results were beginning to appear. It was clear that her body was setting about repairing the nerves, which it felt was the most important thing to do first. The feeling of normality was beginning to return to the leg and she said that she when touching the thigh it felt as though her hand was much closer than on prior occasions. Clearly the healing plasma was repairing the neural network nearer to the skin. Iris was very pleased to tell me that the calf muscle was starting to rebuild. This was amazing to see week by week.

After ten weeks of treatment we had reached the point where obviously the healing plasma was seeping into the heel; it was feeling warmer week by week. Despite the problems with the whole of her leg, the right heel had been the cause of most of her concern, even though discomfort and/or pain was present constantly.

By the twelfth week 'heat' was flowing into her right leg very easily, the whole process was speeding up and the healing plasma was getting into the heel. Iris had previously likened the feeling inside her heel to a peardrop of cold steel. Now the sharp, well defined shape of the peardrop had been worked on and the shape was being broken up. At first the edges of the shape had become 'woolly'. The following week the cold inside feeling of the heel was becoming 'mushy'. Two weeks later the 'heat' had permeated the whole heel and the cold inside had changed. Week by week the heel condition was improving until eventually there was no coldness inside the heel. The whole leg had recovered to almost normality. The heel was normal but there was still an aggravation at the back of the heel. Two more treatments eliminated this and the entire leg was almost normal. The calf muscle was still building and the thigh was still getting very warm. Clearly there was still some work to do to repair the whole of the neural network in the right leg.

In the case of Iris the original back injury had created inflammation around the spine and impeded the neuroflow down through the sciatic nerves. Because the brain did not have full monitoring control over all parts of her right leg, the leg began to suffer. This was because the brain could read the situation beyond the back inflammation and therefore could not instruct the repair and maintenance systems to pay full service to that leg. The longer it went on, the worse the situation became.

Muscles require instruction for control of movement and need to be maintained in a good working condition. The brain controls everything through the peripheral and autonomic nerves. Control is also expected on the maintenance and repair systems that are involved in the renewal of cells and groups of cells, not so much in the division and manufacture of individual cells, but certainly in calling for groups of cells to be replaced and in arranging the disposal of cells. If this is the case, then we can see the brain's involvement in the maintenance of the joints of the body, notably in the lower back and legs. These are the areas with which we generally associate 'arthritis'.

I will now discuss the way in which, I believe, osteo and rheumatic arthritis appear. I remind you of a previous statement in this book, that the body has no language and therefore does not recognise these two 'DISEASES'. The brain controls the body's functions through the nervous system. This is a most important statement to remember.

Any ball joint in the legs, arms and hands, requires constant lubrication. The way in which this happens in the body is for the surfaces of the ball and socket to be lined with what we call cartilage. This is a very tough and gristly type of material. To provide the lubrication, a synovial membrane at the joint edge secretes a frictionless lubricant called synovial fluid, the cells of the synovial fluid slip in between the articulating surfaces of the joint, which permits virtually frictionless movement of the joint. This process cannot be entirely random. There is a mass of nerves at every joint and this applies to the knees in particular. Because of this, there must be a reason for the presence of the cells and I believe that this process is controlled by the brain using the NEUROFLOW along the nerves. When the course of neuroflow is uninterrupted the process of renewal and disposal of the waste material, used cells, etc. runs smoothly. If the course of neuroflow is interrupted the brain is unable to monitor and give instruction for the normal function of the lubrication of the joint and the renewal process in the joint falters. The result is that waste material from dead cells of the lubricant are not washed out. Instead they stay in the area of contact. More cells from the lubricant are issued and come into the contact area and consequently more waste material collects. Eventually, the waste material grows to such an extent that it inhibits the movement of the joint and it begins to feel stiff. After a while the packed cells start to be expelled from the joint simply by the pressure from the incoming cells. The joint feels easier. Eventually, as the whole process continues unabated, the joint becomes so clogged up that the joint starts to grind the waste material into the surfaces of both the ball and the socket and it starts to become inflamed. This process goes on and in due course the surface of the cartilage on both the ball and possibly the socket is breached. This exposes the bone structure behind and the result is that various types of cells from the overall joint mix with the bone cells. This should not happen, as these different cells were never meant to mix, and this foreign mixture then allows in bacteria and viruses. This then is one of the causes of the breakdown of the boney material, hence OSTEOARTHRITIS.

In my clinic I have asked my clients about the chronological events that happened to them before they were diagnosed as having 'arthritis'. In almost all cases, they reported it to me in the following order:

1. Feeling stiff in the lower back in the mornings when getting out of bed. Feeling stiff getting out of and getting into the car. This stiffness feeling would wear off after a short while.
2. Sometime later, the stiffness worsens and the lower back becomes sore and painful.
3. They start to get cramp in the legs.
4. The knees start to give way and then they too begin to hurt.
5. The hips hurt and walking becomes difficult.
6. The pain in the knees and hips become so painful that the doctor diagnose ARTHRITIS.

I believe that this is how arthritis develops:
Normally, the person who has no lower back pain or stiffness at all, or has suffered no injury, will have no pain problem in their legs or hips.

If an intervention problem arises to the sciatic nerves, such as inflammation due to bacteria attack, or some other reason such as pinched nerves or something else (excluding physical damage), then the neuroflow is interrupted, altered or stopped. This small problem, if left unchecked, inevitably grows into something worse. At first, the client may just feel a little twinge or stiffness and they live with it or try to work it off. Working in the gym helps at first but the pain returns at a later date. Sitting in the car becomes a chore. Sitting in a theatre or cinema becomes a problem. The results are that the sufferer starts to shuffle in a theatre seat to the annoyance of others and with considerable discomfort to themselves. Later, the hip starts to hurt and the feet and toes get cold - later still the feet are continuously cold, despite the differences in climate. Then the knees begin to hurt, resulting in an inability to play golf or play with the children or simply bend down any more. Cramp begins to occur, which can be very painful, and so on. This pattern is repeated in this book more than once so as to illustrate the inexorable progress to an inevitable conclusion, ARTHRITIS.

Therefore I believe that arthritis is not really a disease in itself. Rather, it is a condition that is the result of long term deprivation of the brain's neuroflow. I also believe that this applies to some forms of Rheumatoid Arthritis.

If, however, the client asks for treatment from a Reflexologist the repair process is set in motion. When treatment is in process or after the session is finished, the client is in a relaxed state. Being relaxed, the brain is not working on muscular movement; therefore there is no call on the repair system. This allows the treatment to be initiated with greater ease, allowing the full value of the healing process to be carried out without diversion and the client starts to feel a very comforting and warm feeling in the lower back and in the legs. I have noticed in my clinic that initially the warmth appears in one of two ways. In 60% of clients, the first indication of warmth is almost always in the lower back, even though there may be other symptoms in need of attention. The other 40% of clients feel the warmth in their feet first.

I have proposed an answer for this. We know that in times of great stress the body equips itself to deal with the problem by either fighting or by fleeing - the fight or flight situation. When adrenaline is produced by the adrenal glands the body goes into a state of readiness. If the decision is taken to flee, it is no good fleeing unless the body is in a sufficiently good condition to achieve it. When the lower back gets warm very early in the Reflexology treatment, it is because the brain considers it of prime importance to put the lower back into a good condition. This is essential if the person is to run away. Therefore the lower back gets warm first. Should the client have absolutely nothing wrong with the lower back then this situation does not follow. Repeated treatments by a Reflexologist will produce similar results and the client starts to feel progressively more relaxed and comfortable. The client reports that cramp ceases within a few weeks, almost immediately their knees don't hurt so much, their hips are much better, and their back is not so stiff; consequently life becomes brighter and lifting children is now possible without fear of pain. The number of treatments given will vary greatly depending on the severity of the complaint and age of the client. The client often feels that they have taken on a new lease of life. The body has put itself back onto the Lifepath, which is where the client should have been all through their life. The body has been restored according to the standard, making it possible for the Lifepath to be satisfied. Quality of life has been restored and surely, that is what we all seek.

Following each successive treatment, the intensity of the warmth may reduce. The client feels that the body is overcoming the problem. When no warmth at all is felt it indicates that there is no more restoration work to be done by the repair and maintenance system until the next time. So when no warmth at all is experienced, the brain is back in full command of the body, which in this case is the lower back and legs. Pain in the lower back may also be due to the sacro-iliac joint being similarly affected by the interference of the course of the neuroflow to the surrounding area or in the joint. This in itself causes irritation in the joint, even though the synovial fluid is still being supplied to allow movement. Therefore, it can be said that there are two systems at work here, one for the movement and one for the maintenance of the joint surfaces. If the joint surfaces are not being maintained because the neuroflow is impeded, the fact is signalled by pain, which is the body's way of saying that something is wrong. This may also upset the neuroflow through local neuroid joint. This explains why, sometimes, intense heat is felt in the sacrum area, following a Reflexology treatment. This also applies to the muscle structure either side of the sacrum and lumbar sections of the spine. They similarly have suffered with lack of maintenance, hence aching across the lower back. The sacro iliac joint is a major focal point for the movement of the body. It carries a lot of weight, as well as facilitating movement of the legs and hips. The normal working of the joint is essential for these movements. I believe that if there is interruption spanning a number of years, of neuroflow from the brain to the area surrounding the joint, it can result in the degeneration of the lining of the joint. The consequence of this, as with any other joint in the body, will be pain. In addition, the brain uses the surrounding muscles to try to protect the area in pain and these muscles themselves then stiffen. If this condition remains unattended, the muscles receive interrupted neuroflow and they become the cause of pain, in addition to the original problem. The patient is getting further and further away from the Lifepath.

The same can be said about the spine. The nervous system abounds around the spine, keeping it supple and in good condition by ensuring that the waste cell material is disposed of efficiently. An example of the above, in practice, is of a client who had developed painful knees, after having suffered with back ache for many years. She was expecting to develop arthritis, as her mother and grandparents had suffered before her. The bad knees were evidence for her of the inevitability of her fate. Weekly Reflexology treatments produced in the lower back, both legs and particularly the knees, the warmth that I expected. The knees in particular got very 'hot' in the first three weeks of treatment. By the end of the sixth week, the level of warmth in her joints had reduced to a pleasant soft feeling and she was able to resume her sporting activity, albeit slowly. Walking upstairs and downstairs became natural and easy without a thought to her previously painful knees. In fact, she was getting back to her old life. Now she visits me once a month and suffers no more than an occasional pain, just a twinge in her right knee, which is put right when she visits. Every treatment produced a low level of warmth in the right knee and a renewed feeling of comfort. Having had a M.R.I (Magnetic Resonance Imaging) scan, no sign of arthritis could be detected. Her quality of life has been improved. What is more she still has no sign of the genetic arthritis that she dreaded developing in her knees.

Another graphic case adding to the debate, is of a woman who was in great pain. She came to me and said that she had been given a medical diagnosis which stated she had osteoarthritis in the hips and knees. She had reported that her first complaint started with a very painful lower back. She had been to her doctor who prescribed rest and painkillers, which had a marginal effect on her pain, so more powerful painkillers were prescribed. These worked a little better for a while, but their effectiveness, as far as pain reduction was concerned, was diminishing. She was prescribed a total of twelve weeks physiotherapy, at the end of which some relief was experienced but the pain soon returned. By this time she was getting cramp in both legs and her feet were very cold. She was referred to a pain clinic where she said she was offered more painkillers and then an epidural injection. By now her knees were getting bad, they hurt a great deal and her mobility was severely curtailed. She came to me to see if I could do anything to ease the pain. She had been offered 'replacement' knees and hips, but she would have to wait quite some time for this to be done. Surprisingly the X-rays which had been carried out showed that the osteoarthritis was not as bad as first thought.

When she came to me for help I applied a full treatment to both feet, but went back to reinforce the treatment on the reflexes for the lumbar, sacrum and coccyx, plus the reflexes for the sacro iliac joint, sciatic nerve, hip and knee, all of which are concerned with the lower back area. After about twenty minutes her lower back began to warm up, as did her legs and hips. She described her knees as being very hot. After some forty minutes, the intensity of the heat was reducing. When she was about to leave, she reported that her pain level was reduced and she was still warm. Subsequent visits reduced the pain even further until about eight weeks later she told me that she could walk into and around town, do her shopping and then walk home again. She could physically pick up her grandchild much more easily and without fear of dropping the child. Her quality of life improved tremendously. The original deterioration can be clearly seen in the above. Ache in the lower back became worse and worse over the years. Later her hip began to hurt and her foot was always cold. Later still, she got cramp in her calf and thigh muscles and her knee started to hurt. All on the right hand side of her body. If we look at the chronological progression of her developing complaints in reverse, then we have the cold feet, knee, cramp, hip and lower back. It was her knees that she complained about at first. There is progressive activity here. The possibility was that if we could initially have stopped the pain in the lower back, then probably we could have stopped the hip and knee hurting and getting worse. We might also have prevented the cramp. I recall something about great oaks and little acorns!

I recognise that whole industries and charitable organisations exist to help people with arthritis and lower back pain and this has turned into a major expense for these charities and the health services. I also realise that a simple look at these sometimes chronic conditions might seem presumptuous. It may be wondered just how can this simple, proposed theory explain what can be done to prevent arthritis taking a hold on people? Incredible as it may seem, the evidence that I see daily in my clinic leads me to believe that with monthly treatments of Reflexology following an agreed initial course of treatment, it is possible to stave off the ravages of arthritis. It is possible!

It will always be difficult to get away from conventional thinking when considering these conditions. We are locked into procedures that are cast in concrete. When we are in such trouble, it is quite normal for us to visit our doctor. We consider it normal to embark on a course of drug therapy and possibly surgery. This is normal procedure! If we can look away from the end result and instead look back chronologically, as I have advocated time and time again, we may well see the progressive pattern of pain until arthritis was diagnosed. Then ultimately the source of the problem can be traced. We call a condition arthritis when recognised symptoms occur in the body. The body sees the pain only as a pain and information feedback. The body has no name for it. When the body detects something wrong internally through the neural network, it uses the systems at its disposal within the body to fight everything. It cannot bring in outside help by itself. I believe that arthritis is an internal condition. If arthritis is an inside disease - or maladjustment then it should be seen in that light. If it is the result of something going badly wrong, not something brought in from outside then it should be seen in that light.

Accidental damage to the legs and lower back may turn into arthritis, because the local nerve system is damaged and thus the service of neuroflow to that area, therefore the monitoring ability of the brain, is interrupted. The maintenance system will attempt to effect a repair. If successful, the area of the injury returns to normal. If not, then the problems progressively worsens. If the injury is too much for the body to repair by itself, a reflexologist can assist and persuade the body to have a go at a repair. Over many treatments, surprising results may well be accomplished. Complete recovery cannot be guaranteed, but an improvement in the situation may well be achieved.

It cannot be said too often that keeping the nerves in good condition by receiving Reflexology treatments will be worthwhile in the long run. I am often asked if I can do anything about arthritis. I have to say that it depends on the severity of the complaint. If the condition has progressed too far and joint replacement is not only being considered but is actually necessary, Reflexology cannot recoup the situation. However, it can reduce the pain level and give some measure of comfort. It is only where the condition has not gone too far that reversal becomes possible.

Neck, Arms and Hands - Arthritis
The human body has evolved to give us an upright stance so our two legs have become longer and stronger, whilst our two arms have evolved into the shorter and more workable limbs that they now are. The nerves in the neck that exit at the cervical part of the spine (neck) proceed down the arms to the hands. The names of the nerves down the arm are various and it is a complicated distribution network. For our purposes we know that there is a direct link between the brain and the fingertips. All nerves are connected to other nerves but all arrive at the cervical spine.

The same problems that occur in the legs also appear in the arms, except that in this case the spinal connection is from the cervical section of the spine. The neck is a very flexible limb and is moving almost constantly. The same can be said about the arms and certainly the hands. The need for constant renewal of cells and lubrication in the neck, shoulder, elbow, wrist and fingers, is equally important.

We start to experience a stiff neck, perhaps from the way we sleep or perhaps following a previous motor accident from which whiplash develops some months, or even years later. Bad posture can also be the root cause when we find it difficult to turn the head. Our shoulders soon begin to ache, then we become aware of our arms, the hands begin to tingle and the elbow hurts. The hands get cold and the fingers begin to hurt. Ultimately, arthritis appears in the fingers. Depending on the length of time the condition has existed and what part of the brachial nerve system has been affected, the shoulder may become 'frozen', the elbow may also be affected. Pain is not nice but it must be remembered that pain is the brain's way of telling us something is wrong. The fingers and elbows swell and life quality is drastically reduced. Medication is taken and sometimes an injection or two are offered.

The longer these problems are left unattended the worse they become and the more difficult they are to eliminate. Then we are into a holding situation where pain can be reduced and controlled, but that is all as the root cause of the problem is not being tackled. Where arthritis is confirmed following medical diagnosis, the body cannot recover the Lifepath to its fullest extent. The brain cannot read the situation locally due to the inflammation further back in the arm or neck. Surgical intervention may then be the only course open to the client. We are then into replacement of shoulders and elbows. By applying Reflexology through a trained and fully qualified therapist who belongs to a recognised association, much can be done to improve the nation's health and improve an individual client's lifestyle.

The following illustrates the progression of pain yet again and the accompanying damage to the limb(s) if the first signs of pain are ignored. A case is recalled here where a man came to the clinic following advice from his wife. He complained of painful hands and fingers and, on examination, I found that the fingers were unable to close on the palms of each hand, nor could they be opened. They were completely fixed. The hands and fingers were swollen and the skin was white, shiny and taught. His shoulders and neck had been stiff and painful for some months before coming to see me. Now his elbows started to get painful; two months previously his hands had started to swell and the fingers became fixed. He was very distressed complaining that he could not do anything. His hands were useless and the pain was terrible. His wife had told me that he was a bit impatient and was looking for miracles straight away. I had to tell him right at the beginning that results could not be guaranteed and the process of recovery, to whatever level might be possible, would be long into the year. It was then March 1996. He overcame his disappointment and agreed to carry on to the end, after all he had no prospect of recovery from conventional medicine. However this should not to be interpreted as a criticism of conventional medicine.

Treatment commenced that March. The weather was very cold and my client was matching it with his demeanour. He told me that he tried to hand dry some dishes at home that morning but had dropped the first plate, which only served to show him how bad the condition was. Over the first two weeks, I gave him an overall Reflexology treatment over both feet, this elicited extreme pain from the reflexes for the neck, cervical spine, shoulder girdles and shoulder joints, arms, elbows and hands. I had to strike a balance between inflicting extreme pain on his feet to achieve a quicker response and ensuring that the body would produce the healing response during the treatment session. I expected the healing response to become noticeable by the patient, in line with my working theory and I did not tell the client what to expect as I wanted him to tell me what he was experiencing. By the end of the third treatment, the client was beginning to "feel as though there was an electric fire next to his neck, because it felt as though it was burning". A few minutes later, he said that his shoulders were beginning to feel warm. He was showing some sign of anxiety at this point, so I felt compelled to tell him what, (in my opinion), was happening to him. Once he realised that this was nothing more than a natural process, he was much happier and was keen to report further on what he felt. He said that he could feel the warmth spreading from his neck and across his shoulder on both sides. After a few more minutes he said that both his arms were warm but the elbows were hot. Last of all, his hands began to feel warm. After a full forty minutes, he was experiencing a comfortable 'glowing' feeling from his neck down to his fingers. He looked disbelieving but grateful because at last he was more comfortable than when he came in and was now without pain. He said, "It is not possible for you to fully appreciate the pleasure that I am feeling. Just to be without pain even for only a few minutes was worth a king's ransom." He looked very happy. At the end of the treatment on that third week, I told him about my theory and how I thought it was affecting him. He is an intelligent man and although he did not fully understand what I was saying, he did agree that something was going on inside him and he was still feeling the warmth in his neck. I told him that experience had shown me that the pain would return, although I could not say when, but it might not be quite so painful. He left my clinic a happier man.

The fourth week produced the same healing response as the previous week. The client was expecting it to happen, and it did, but much quicker this time. I could argue that his body was expecting it to happen and it was all a question of mind over matter, however, I did not think so because the healing response became apparent only after the treatment was given in session, otherwise he would have felt warm as soon as he sat down, or elsewhere, but he did not. Gradually, his neck began to warm up and his hands started to tingle. By now, the hands were beginning to become very warm. At the end of the fourth treatment he was starting to move his head a little more than before.

When he arrived on the fifth week he reported that his neck was much easier now and he could turn it through 180°, but he was anxious to get on with his hands. That week's treatment, as in all previous weeks, was centred on the prominent reflexes, which were the neck, cervical spine, shoulder girdles and joints, arms, elbows and hands. The full treatment was carried out after the specific treatment to these reflexes. This was to enable the healing process to start at the earliest possible time. The pattern of travel by the healing plasma was clearly experienced by the patient, in that he could feel the warmth starting in his neck, moving across the shoulders and down the arms. Each nerve has its own blood supply and the healing plasma runs in the body through the circulation system. The healing plasma is leaked out to the nerve and starts its cleaning and repairing process. This induces the glowing feeling but is more simply experienced by the client as feeling warm. This pattern followed the same routine for the next few weeks and by the sixth week the client reported that his shoulders were feeling much better and he could move them without pain. However, he still had pain in the arms and hands. Overall, the level of intensity of pain had reduced, and the treatment progressed with little obvious gains being achieved. At every single treatment, the client experienced the same warm feeling running from his neck down to his fingers. By the eighth week, he reported that his elbows were hurting less, and his neck and shoulders continued to give no pain. This did not deter him from pressing me for some improvement in the hands. I had to tell him again that it was his body's own choice to dictate the order in which reclamation took place. Obviously, the body could not get at the hands until the neck, shoulder, elbow and arm had been dealt with which cleared the way, so allowing the healing plasma to inch its way forward until it reached the hands. It was noted that the hands had been warm at every treatment, but the neck had been warmest. His hands would surely come last in the line. Thinking about this further, the hand can work only if the forearm is able to create the correct motive power and direction. The forearm can work only if the elbow and upper arm are in a healthy enough state to provide the same correct motive power and direction, and similarly the upper arm and elbow can work only if the shoulder and neck can provide the necessary motive power and direction. None of the individual parts of the arm will allow the hand to work, unless they themselves can perform their function in combination with the adjacent part. So the healing process first reclaims the neck, then the shoulder girdle and joint, upper arm, elbow and forearm.

My client followed the essence of what he was told, even if not the letter, but still wanted to get his hands moving again. By the twelfth treatment session he was still getting warm from his neck, down both arms to his fingertips. He was not only getting warm but he was also getting an increased amount of tingling in both hands. It indicated that more of the healing plasma was being applied to the locally damaged nerve system and this was causing the tingling. This was good news for both of us. By now, he had full use restored to both of his arms up to and including his neck. He reported no pain apart from his hands. He left me that week forgetful of the work that had been achieved so far but saying that at last his hands were getting some attention. The following three weeks saw the same healing process as had happened in the twelfth week, but on the sixteenth week we started to see a change take place in his hands. It seemed unimportant to my client but I was quite excited by it. From the first week that I saw this client I could see that the colour and texture of the skin on his neck and whole arms were what I would think of as normal for a man of his age. The exceptions were the hands, which as I described earlier, were immovable and the skin was taut, white and swollen. The skin had an appearance of tight latex that had been waxed. This appearance was from the fingers and tops of the hands up to and including the wrists. This week it was different. This week I could actually see the normal textured skin of his forearm begin to creep over the wrists and replace the waxed swollen look that they had shown from the first week of treatment. It was just as though the body was reclaiming the hands. I do not mean to imply that I saw this event in action, but I had noted it from the previous week. My client was less appreciative of the importance of the process but he was beginning to recognise the progress he had made. The next three weeks saw more progress in his hands. His normal skin texture and colour had encroached onto his hands up to the start of the fingers and the swelling had gone from where the normal skin had reached. The fingers had all begun to get very warm, as had the rest of the arms, shoulders and neck, however, he could feel shooting pains going down into the fingers. I believe that this signified that the neuroflow from the brain was attempting to regain control. The twentieth week saw the fingers begin to be reclaimed by the normal skin and in addition, the client was able to move his fingers a little. Each treatment produced the same warmth, indicating that the healing process was working. The twenty first, twenty second and twenty third treatments saw the client improving each week. The twenty fourth treatment came and the client reported that his fingers were now working so well that at last he could do things again. In fact, he had indeed got the movement and freedom from pain that he wanted in all the body structure from his neck down to his fingers. His fingers could now move well but could not straighten out too much; even so, the movement that was possible was almost normal. The hands looked normal as far as appearance was concerned and he said he could now dry the dishes without dropping them. How our needs and perspectives change with age. He could now put on his own coat without help and do up the buttons by himself and he could now drive the car safely. The list was endless, but the greatest thing he wanted to do was to get back to his garden.

This client came back to see me occasionally to keep himself up to par, and he has done very well. The knuckles on both hands still look slightly enlarged and after more treatment I could see that surprisingly the size of the knuckles was reducing. Even later still, his knuckles are almost normal and full movement was now possible. I am sure that this man's symptoms would have turned into full-blown osteoarthritis. As it is, this client is back in the mainstream of life and is very happy for it.

This sort of case does make me think that there is a standard against which all body parts and functions have to be measured and the purpose is to meet the requirements for the Lifepath. This case clearly shows what nasty things can arise as a result of not dealing with small problems at an early stage. After some weeks of treatment, his neck became much looser and he could move his head without pain or difficulty. His elbows started to hurt more but his hands were beginning to warm up, and later his shoulders stopped hurting and he could now put on his own coat. The elbows stopped hurting and the swelling on the hands began to slowly reduce. Each treatment was progressive and eventually the fingers showed signs of movement. Up to the time of writing he still has no pain in his neck, shoulders or elbows, and his hands are gradually returning to normal. The amazing thing was that the unusual appearance of the skin on the backs of his hands began to diminish with the normal skin appeaarance spreading from the wrists, back over the knuckles, reclaiming lost ground. This man no longer takes medication under the advice of his doctor. His is very pleased with his progress. If we leave these problems then the end result may turn into arthritis, which I believe is not really a disease, but a condition.

Sports Injuries
Related to this chapter, we can look a little at some of the things that afflict those who practise one or more sports. Common among the problems which are frequently highlighted by the media are things such as pulled hamstrings, cramp, damage to achilles tendon and lower back pain. None of these problems is good news to an athlete. Most of those who suffer would consult a physiotherapist or sports doctor in a sports clinic and possibly will then be given a muscle massage. There is much technology now available in such clinics, most of which

may be helpful, but if the problem is repeated and becoming too frequent, especially at the wrong times when the athlete least needs it, then something else needs to be done. Reflexology is the way back to athletic health. Instead of relying just on exercise, a much speedier recovery can be expected with the help of Reflexology.

Bearing in mind all that has been said earlier in this book concerning the healing plasma and how this material must be circulating in the body constantly, it is possible to look at the effect on the body by doing exercise or training. If a person has been swimming or running for example, the physical structure of the body needs not only oxygen and nutrients, but also requires that all joints and muscles are kept lubricated and in pace with the activity being undertaken. There will be an ever increasing demand by the extra work loaded on the body, for the products contained in the healing plasma, produced by the adrenal glands. This may also be relevant to injuries that athletes seem to acquire after the first few years of trouble free activity. It may be that the call on the body to produce so much healing plasma for the servicing of the body structure increases with the age of the person and the increase of body mass. There must come a time when all possible production of healing plasma is being used to service the body that is being trained so there is not much left over for the servicing of the parts that become extended beyond 'normal' activity, for example, in a race. The fact that intensive training has produced a dramatic increase in body mass does not mean that the systems which maintain the body also grow. They may well stay the same size, but only enough for the body that it was intended to serve as per the genetic blueprint. The explosion of effort in a short race puts such an enormous strain on things like hamstrings and achilles tendons that there may not be enough natural healing plasma to cope. This may well explain why a perfectly fit athlete suddenly pulls up in a race with hamstring or achilles tendon pain. It may also explain why athletes who continue to train to get through the problem, actually take a lot longer than might be thought necessary to return to the track or field. Sometimes, after such an injury, some athletes never seem to quite achieve what was possible prior to the injury.

Chapter 8

Circulation

Chapter four has already touched on this subject and references to this chapter have been made elsewhere in these pages. Expanding on the idea that the body systems work hand in glove with each other, apply your thoughts to not just a part the mechanical components of the system, such as the heart, veins, pulmonary arteries, etc., but look at why the system exists at all as a whole. The body needs to pump blood around the system to supply the tissue structure with necessities such as oxygen, nutrients, macrophages, lymphocytes, other products of the immune system and all products of the repair system. It also carries the cell debris collected by the capillaries and by the lymphatic system which has been deposited into the blood circulation system via the lymph nodes. The blood is then filtered by the liver making waste material ready for elimination.

To enable the distribution of the blood around the body, a distribution network of blood vessels is used. The arteries carry blood from the heart. They get smaller and smaller until they become tiny, but are still made the same way as the larger arteries. The smallest of these are called arterioles. Each has a cross sectional view which shows four layers of material in the wall of the tube. One layer that appears in both arterioles, arteries and veins, is a layer of smooth muscle. As previously said, muscle has no intelligence and there seems to be little purpose for its presence in the tubing of the blood vessels if it were it not for the fact that very small filament nerves are attached to the smooth muscle throughout the vascular system. Therefore a direct route to the brain is established, which enables the brain to control a particular section of any blood vessel at will, even at the extremities of the body where the feet, toes, hands and fingers are located. The neuroflow from the brain keeps open these arterioles by stimulating the smooth muscle in the wall of the blood vessel. This stimulation excites the smooth muscle and it stretches to its maximum length, creating a maximum diameter in that part of the blood vessel under control of that particular nerve. By doing this the maximum quantity of blood flows through the maximum bore, which maintains the pressure against the wall of the blood vessel and keeps it within the required parameters for the rest of the body. This phenomenon also explains how the body can seem to direct blood etc., here, there and everywhere, whenever it is needed. It simply stops exciting a small section of blood vessel so that it collapses, almost, and stops the blood going through that route, therefore it must go the other route that leads to the injury site.

If a problem happens in the neck (see Chapter 6), then the neuroflow coursing down the nervous system to the arterioles in the fingers is interrupted. The smooth muscle in the arterioles does not receive the complete neuroflow. The part of the smooth muscle in the blood vessel that is controlled by the filament nerve, which is not receiving full neuroflow, does not know what to do and it partially or sometimes completely collapses. This restricts the flow of blood into the feet and hands and there is just enough to keep operating the primary functions such as care of skin, tissue and nails, etc. The one component missing is body heat. The smaller volume of blood flowing in the feet and hands means that any body heat it did carry was dissipated before the blood reached the feet. The feet and hands get cold because there is not enough caloric value (heat) in the blood. If the lack of blood is long term the skin may suffer due to lack of nutrients. It is an essential function of the blood that it carries heat around the body. If the blood flow is reduced then the calorific value of the blood is also reduced, thus the flesh does not warm up sufficiently and extremities become colder than normal. I believe that the start of this decline of heat transfer is the lack of neuroflow through the filament nerves connected to the smooth muscle in the blood vessels. Even then, the start of the problem may be further back than that. After all, what caused the interference of the neuroflow in the first place?

When Reflexology is applied, the 'healing plasma' is distributed into the leg or arm via the blood circulation system and coats the nerves that require attention, as they may require extensive repair throughout a limb, which in due course, will make the arm or leg feel warm. After a while, the hands and feet appear to the client to be warm but if touched the flesh on both hands and feet will feel as cold as they usually do, even though they apparently feel warm. A little while later, the nerves attached to the arterioles receive the correct neuroflow and they distend the walls of the blood vessels. By stimulating the smooth muscle to the correct diameter the full flow of blood resumes and brings with it more body heat. It is at that point that the flesh of the hands and feet start to feel physically warm. The increase of blood flow brings with it an increase of body heat which is transferred by conduction, to the surrounding tissue. Even after only one treatment many people go home with very warm feet and hands. The first awareness of heat in the hands or feet may be quite marked, even though the extremities still feel cold to the touch. This is clear evidence that something else is warming up or appearing to feel warm. The healing plasma is working on the nerve in a chemical or molecular way. It does this to clean and repair the nerve so that it is ready for transmission of neuroflow at the correct rate. It is only later that the hands or feet actually feel warm to the touch.

In my opinion this clearly demonstrates how closely linked the neurological system and the circulation system are. Breaking new ground is a lonely business but I was most encouraged by some information, which had been sent to me by a good friend who was aware of my theories. This paper was compiled by Salvador Moncada, M.D, F.R.S, and Annie Higgs, M.Sc, and appeared in The New

England Journal of Medicine of December 30th 1993 (Ref.1). By chance, this paper has found a home with my theories. The work concerned, "The L-ARGININE-NITRIC OXIDE PATHWAY" describes the presence of Nitric Oxide (NO) in the body and the search for a role for it in the body. I have attempted to paraphrase this paper in one respect only. The authors clearly see the use of NO in the body in an ever-increasing dimension and the paper talks about the NO being used as a means of carrying messages to and from the neuro transmitters and being present in the smooth muscle of the vascular system.

The authors make the case for a connection between the action of the NO in the blood vessel wall and HYPERTENSION. I suggest that NO is a messenger bearing data from the various function centres in the brain via neuro flow to their destination. This is the means whereby the brain stimulates the smooth muscle in the wall of the blood vessel. If the passage of the NO is impeded then stimulation takes places to a lesser degree. Hence the wall of a blood vessel collapses. The flow of blood reduces and the pressure against the wall of the blood vessel upstream of the blockage increases, resulting in HYPERTENSION. The appearance of the feet and hands can sometimes appear blue in colour. This is said to be cyanosis, after the colour cyan. This is because the deoxygenated blood is very slow to move away so the predominant colour is dark red (a little bit blue).When the full operational condition in the sciatic and brachial nerve systems is restored, the colour of both feet and hands improve, thus visually telling the client that things are getting back to normal.

Let us go on one step further. Reynaud's Syndrome is where the flesh of the toes, or more commonly the fingers, takes on a whitened appearance. Oxygenated blood has been prevented from entering the digits whilst the deoxygenated blood is prevented from escaping the tissue, leaving the flesh the colour of almost white. The client always reports that the fingers and feet are very cold. It is the blood that changes the colour to what we call flesh colour. In the case of Reynaud's Syndrome, the arterioles have closed almost completely at the entry to those digits. When Reflexology is applied, the healing plasma seeks out and repairs the interruption to the neuroflow, both in the digit or maybe further up the arm or even in the neck. By the restoration of the brachial and sciatic systems to full operational condition, the blood again flows into the fingers or toes, warming them up and changing their colour to that of normal flesh.

To illustrate this, a series of treatments was given to a woman for a certain problem, however that particular problem is not the subject of what we are covering here. She complained also of a white and numb third toe on the right foot, and similarly she had a white third toe on the left foot. Treatment of the sciatic nerve and associated sacrum spine reflexes, sacro-iliac joint and knee reflexes made both her legs become warm. The warmth travelled down from her back and reached her foot and lastly her toes. We both watched her white toe slowly change colour to match the colour of the adjacent toes. It felt very warm to my touch and also to the patient. This all happened on the first treatment and it was interesting to note that the only two related areas that were warm in her body were the toe and the lower back.

A man who had damage to his shoulder found he had lost mobility in his arm and the hand was blue in colour and cold. Treatment showed a marked improvement in his arm mobility and his hand was warmer with a better colour. By applying Reflexology the circulation system is improved. This brings more blood, more oxygen, more body heat and more body nutrients to the site of any injury. The body's own maintenance and repair systems are afforded much better access via the upgraded neural network and the client feels better.

'Varicose Veins Here' is part of a Question and Answer article which was written by John Campbell, RMN,RGN. Dip.Nursing, B.A.. It appeared in the Nursing Times, February 3rd 1993, Volume 89, No.5

Q. What types of shock are primarily caused by low peripheral resistance ?

A. Neurogenic shock (originating in the central nervous system) may occur in patients who are in pain; also in patients with brain and spinal injuries. Injuries of the central nervous system may cause inhibition of the sympathetic nerves [Passmore, Robson, J.S.(eds). A Companion Guide To Medical Studies (vol.3). Oxford: Blackwell, 1975]. This effect reduces cardiac activity and the upshot is vasodilation. Both of these effects will reduce blood pressure.

Varicose Veins
Of each of the people coming into my clinic with this complaint, I have asked if they have currently, or have suffered in the past, with a bad back. This may have been in the form of pain or stiffness. The vein has a thinner tube wall than the artery. The veins in the legs also have smooth muscle as part of the structure. To this smooth muscle filament nerves are connected in the same way as for the arteries. I believe that if the neuroflow to the particular section of smooth muscle is interrupted then, at a certain point, the vein may close enough to allow only some blood through and at the same time pressure will build up behind the restriction.

I have concluded that this causes the vein, up stream of the constriction, to laterally expand and subsequently swell. This is because a vein has a thinner wall structure than an artery and cannot resist for long the pressure exerted upon it. This leads to the appearance of what we call a varicose vein. Again, the interruption of the neuroflow will normally be near the vein and possibly due to local damage. I have examined quite a few clients with varicose veins. In some of these cases the veins gave the appearance of being very long in structure and it was established that somewhere upstream of the vein, damage could be accounted for due to a knock, or even a bad back. This meant neuroflow impedance had occurred and would seem to go some way in support of my conclusions.

I have not been able to see if it is possible to reverse the mis-shapen vein, but Reflexology will very likely stop the condition worsening. If treatment is given before the problem gets too bad, it may well stop the condition occurring in the first place. This is by far the most desirable situation.

I have heard some people tell me that they have had bad pains in their legs and they were advised to have their veins 'stripped'. I have gleaned much information from my clients and formed the conclusions I have stated above. I can therefore provide an acceptable explanation as to why it is that even after veins have been stripped, the client still has pain in the legs. It is my belief that the original problem may well have been impeded neuroflow to the affected veins, which if so, could well have been corrected by using Reflexology and effecting a repair. This would have reduced the pain and the client would have kept their veins. There will always be people who really do need this operation, but they must surely be small in number. In my opinion, for the vast majority of people an operation of this nature is not always necessary.

The Heart

I have always regarded the heart as a 'stand alone' organ. That was until a woman patient came to see me about the Rheumatoid Arthritis in her shoulders and arms. She had been coming to the clinic for a number of weeks, during which time she had improved considerably and this visit was no exception to any other she had made. She sat in my treatment chair and I proceeded with the session. Having treated both feet, I rested and she reported warmth in her neck and shoulders, which was quite normal. After a minute or so she reported that she was feeling warmth coming down from her neck inside her chest centrally. This was inexplicable because I had not been told about any problem that would indicate this reaction. A moment or two later, she said, with a smile on her face, that her heart palpitations had stopped. Palpitations? What palpitations? Only then did she tell me that she experienced them often. So much so that she tended to ignore them, as she had done so on that occasion and every time that she had attended for treatment. Her palpitations, she reported, had stopped completely. They have not reappeared since.

The nerves from the cardiac ganglion have inputs into the heart structure via filament nerves. The heart, anatomically speaking, is no more than a muscle; therefore the brain must be stimulating the heart in a similar manner as it does any other muscle. The sino-atrial and atrial ventricular nodes provide the impetus that produces the beat. Therefore the neuroflow acts as trigger to the nodes. The heart has a number of filament nerves feeding into it from the autonomic nervous system via the ganglia, and in this case, the warmth (the effect of the healing plasma) had followed the nerves from the neck to one or more ganglia, repairing the impedance (inflammation) that was stopping the full neuroflow between the heart and the brain. This had allowed the brain to see past the inflammation and recognise that there was a problem and it immediately called upon the adrenal glands to produce the healing plasma. This was then directed up to the spine (cervical area) in the neck and followed the nerve to the ganglia and then on to the heart. Consequently the client felt warmth in her neck and on the front (inside) of her central upper chest.

In her case the body had done much to rectify the pain due to the rheumatoid arthritis, and at that session her brain had then been able to see past the inflammation and assess the state of the heart's physical condition. I surmised that the node (Sino-atrial node and Atrioventricular node) looks after the beat of the heart and no more. The heart itself as a structure needs the normal application of the healing plasma that the brain affords to the rest of the body. This stabilises its structure to given parameters (provided by the standard in the brain) thus providing the correct environment within which the heartbeat can be carried out. Under normal circumstances, the heart beats within this framework without problem. If the neuroflow to and from the heart is impeded, then the structure of the heart is destabilised or it grows larger. Depending on the length of time and the severity of the impedance, this could result in palpitations. It may also account for when the heart skips a beat. As far as I am aware, my client has suffered no palpitations since that day.

I began to think about other heart difficulties. The healing plasma in the above case was able to repair the nerve structure and allow the neuroflow route to be reinstated. If this happened for this client, why should it not do the same for more severe heart 'diseases'? I decided to ask a few clients about any relations in their families who had heart problems or who had died from a heart problem. I was astonished to find that of the people who could give me concrete information, on heart problems in their families all reported that their relatives had been treated for (or had not been treated for but nonetheless suffered from) a painful neck and left shoulder. To date, I have established that thirty four people have confirmed the same information. Only two people said that they did not have any neck problem at all, but when I tested their reflexes for the neck, pain was evident. This clearly indicated that a problem was present in their necks but it did not seem apparent to them.

I attended a course in London and a presenter of one of the modules was a nurse. She told me that her husband had died from a heart attack. I asked if she minded talking about the incident and she agreed willingly. Her nursing training came in useful here and I asked if her husband had ever suffered from a neck problem. She told me that he had suffered a really terrible time with a painful neck up to the time of death. She said that she had told the doctor that, in her opinion, the neck was a contributory factor in the case but had been told that this was not so. She remained unconvinced. I told her what I had found and that I was becoming convinced that indeed the bad neck might well have been the starting point for neuroflow deprivation. This would have denied the proper instructions to the heart in a massive way. It may have been this way in her husband's case. She was very interested in what I told her and seemed more than a little relieved to hear someone else explain what she felt.

I attended a meeting in Birmingham, England, and I got talking to a man and his wife about various matters. I was told by the wife that her husband had suffered a heart attack and had been medically supervised ever since. I gently asked if he minded talking about it. He said he was pleased to do so and I asked him if ever he had suffered any form of neck or shoulder trouble prior to his heart attack. He looked at me and said that he had got spondylosis in his neck and suffered a great deal. This pattern was becoming more than coincidental.

We know that people suffer from aortic embolisms, narrowing of the arteries, angina, heart failure, etc. We are presented with scare stories to change our way of life in the good cause of better health. I have defended this approach, but we know that, excepting those who are grossly obese, heart disease affects thin people, fit people, those in a normal state of health as well as overweight people. Why? Could it be that the common cause of many of the heart difficulties which affect us could be due to something so simple as I have related above? I have asked thirty four people so far, if they or their spouses or partners, who had either died or survived a heart attack, had ever suffered with any neck and/or shoulder problems on the left hand side. Up to this point, I have found that one person did not know, one person was not sure, but thirty two people confirmed that this had been the case. In some cases the victim was being treated in hospital for this very complaint. This could not be a coincidence. This might well be the answer as to why such a variant of victims suffer heart attacks even when they are 'fit' and have followed the normal advice of living a healthy lifestyle. So perhaps the precursor to having a heart attack is neither being overweight or not getting enough exercise, it may simply be that a severe neck/shoulder pain on the left side, existed for a period of time and that was sufficient time to create impedance. This is enough of an impedance on the autonomic nerves leading down to the heart, to prevent the brain from seeing that the heart needs the maintenance it should normally be given, so it deteriorates.

Over a period of time the heart deteriorates so much that it finally alerts us to the fact. At first, the client might feel the heart missing a beat and/or racing, then later, angina and then perhaps a heart attack. If the heart does not receive its normal quota of healing plasma, then it will do what all muscles do and stiffen to a greater or lesser degree. The wall of the heart is normally well maintained and it is in constant contact with the brain. It is supple enough to absorb some of the heartbeat provided by the sino nodes. Then it flexes back to create the actual pumping action. Should the heart stiffen slightly, the beat occasionally bounces a little. If the heart wall stiffens a little more, then the beat is bounced more frequently and each beat is reflected before the next one and so it goes faster and faster. When the heart wall stiffens so much, it goes into cramp. Most people know what cramp in the calf muscles feels like. It is very painful, so it is with heart cramp (heart attack), only this can be fatal. This is why thin people as well as overweight people can develop a heart attack. The method of delivering Reflexology that I have developed has produced the rush of healing plasma in the neck of patients and in the upper chest. Before the above knowledge came to me, the significance of this had not been clear. Now it is.

Rethinking Reflexology   by   John C F Moorhouse

Chapter 9

Blood Pressure

I attended a seminar in London for Reflexologists some time ago where a variety of topics were discussed. One of the speakers was a psychologist who had co-operated with two therapists and together, carried out a treatment programme on elderly people who lived at a residential home. No drugs were given. The idea was to establish what benefit, if any, could be given by the treatment with various therapies to individual clients. The psychologist was Dr Sidney Jones who oversaw the whole project. He said at the seminar that almost all patients had responded positively and that he was amazed to find that many of the problems that seem to bother elderly patients had been reduced. He told those who attended that he was so impressed with the results that he himself had signed on for training to become a Reflexologist, and he pleaded that if anyone present could tell him how it worked he would be most grateful. At that time, no such explanation was forthcoming. I was sitting in the audience and bursting to tell him my theory, but I was not ready. The information in this book should now go a long way to satisfying his request.

The problem with hypertension (high blood pressure) is that it cannot be verified by X-ray (only some of the effects can be seen) and it does not show up on an ultra sound picture. Magnetic Resonance Imaging (M.R.I) cannot see it, yet blood pressure is an integral component in the working of our body systems. The only way to detect it is by means of a blood pressure measuring device.

Many recurring comments in the report by Dr. Jones concern blood pressure. In all cases blood pressure was measured and seen to be down from the hypertensive state that existed prior to the commencement of treatment, and this fact went right across the board. Why? What was happening? Doctors will nearly always explain this away by saying that this or that treatment gave the patient relaxation and it is that treatment which reduces blood pressure. Of course, after a Reflexology treatment most people will feel very relaxed. That is not in doubt, but according to the report why is it that after a course of treatment the client's blood pressure apparently falls.

Our bodies are a miracle of design. Charles Darwin wrote about evolution and how he theorised we all evolved from the swamp. We are asked to accept that by a miraculous series of chances we arrived at the state that we are now. This may be the case, but when we ponder the complexity of our bodies it is very hard not to think of ourselves as being designed. If we have been designed, could it have been by Mother Nature or by God's hand? Whoever it was, they had the foresight to include in our bodies' systems, the sole purpose, which is to help us keep free from illness and disease. Our bodies perform repairs on our skin when it breaks and repair other parts of our bodies when they go wrong. In fact, these systems should keep us in good health and free from pain from birth until death. It is an absolutely wonderful plan to provide our bodies with a self repairing structure that can repel invaders.

The main intervention has been the human race itself. We are prisoners of our own existence and, to a large extent, we have attempted to ignore our own defences, substituting them with man made products. Perhaps this is because of the training that medical people are given. They seem to look at the body from one direction only but, as Reflexologists, we look at the same anatomy and physiology that doctors see, but from a different angle. The only fight against hypertension has been to reduce it with drugs after it has been diagnosed. It is only then that we have, or are deemed to have, contracted hypertension. It may not be known how many years prior to the diagnosis of the condition, high blood pressure had been present Under current medical procedures this cannot be answered. It is a common fact in both men and women that as we get older our blood pressure rises.

Because so many people gain weight and do less and less exercise and are diagnosed as having hypertension, they have all been linked together. We have assumed that if you have one problem (say you are overweight) then you are almost certainly going to get the other (hypertension). Looked at in this light, no wonder we are all scared into reducing weight and taking more exercise, neither of which is a bad idea for the overall welfare of the individual, but we are also told that this will reduce blood pressure. When the numbers of people who have hypertension and who also are overweight are so overwhelming, the inference drawn is perhaps understandable. The need to keep blood pressure down is undeniable. With hypertension we are in danger, though not 100% sure, of developing strokes, heart attacks and other complaints, and perhaps much more is affected than we are currently aware.

A great industry has grown up around heart and circulation. The healthcare authorities are always looking for ways to head off future financial expenditure by prevention at an earlier stage. This is a good system. One way is to detect and reduce an individual's blood pressure. The fact is that even with this regime in place, the doctors' surgeries are kept very busy. In hospitals, whole departments are created with their own hierarchy to meet this need, which involves survival after heart attacks or related problems. It is certain that even now, we cannot be certain of the extent of damage caused by hypertension. Complete seminars are given over to discussion of the subject.

The nation's health bill is rising to astronomical heights; so much so, that it seems that healthcare is being rationed in an effort to spend money 'wisely'. Privately run healthcare organisations exercise restraint on future spending commitments by a pricing mechanism, which ensures that they do not accept for membership those with a history of hypertension or heart related diseases. This is a commercially prudent thing to do, but it is left to the state run health authorities to deal with everyone else.

So everyone is constantly seeking ways to reduce that burden and one way is to have a first strike policy. Because so many people are being diagnosed as hypertensive the resultant cost of this diagnosis is rising all the time. Doctors are being advised by manufacturers of new products to reduce hypertension. From this ever increasing range of available products, and based on information from the pharmaceutical company together with personal experience or on experiences from colleagues, a judgement is made and a doctor will prescribe. Sometimes several types of drugs are tried before one is found that is 'suitable', and even then this may result in the client experiencing some unpleasant side affects. Finally one is selected and prescribed.

Once this happens, the client is invariably advised that the tablets must now be taken for life. The patient is now on the hypertensive merry-go-round. They now become a statistic for the marketing plans of the future by the manufacturer of the tablet. No wonder the market for clinical drugs is so huge. In addition, there are other costs that form part of the future spending commitments of charities and social services operated by government. Hospitals will need more expensive equipment to cope with the increasing results of heart and circulation problems. The resulting power of money in these circumstances is awesome, all because we develop hypertension. Obviously something needs to be done so let us get back to the start of the problem. Our bodily systems are configured to help us achieve things at a basic level, the standard. To run, stand up and move our limbs, to the point of contortion for some, we need our organs to work at the correct performance level. We have also been given the ability to react quickly in time of danger or where courage is required. This is all necessary for our own survival. We have a primal instinct for this and to enable it to happen the body must first be put into a state of readiness. In times of great stress, the kidney produces Renin which joins the blood stream. This is a perfectly normal function. Renin combines with a substance produced by the liver and this produces angiotensin. This material causes the blood vessels to constrict and raises the pressure of the blood against the walls of the blood vessels. All this happens quite naturally. By constricting the blood vessels and raising the blood pressure, the speed of the blood through the arteries is increased. This makes it possible for the muscles demand for more oxygen, when in motion, to be met very quickly. The heart begins to pump faster and the lungs operate faster, forcing faster breathing, so that the oxygen in the blood is at a greater concentration and must be delivered by the blood at an increased rate. It can be therefore be appreciated that a rise in blood pressure is a necessary natural function. Clinicians have seen this as the culprit. They tend to use drugs that act upon the kidneys to stop Renin being produced, thus reducing blood pressure. On the whole they seem to work, but all packs of tablets contain warnings about side effects, which in itself appears to indicate that the tablets are not doing the job completely satisfactorily. If they were, there would be no side effects at all.

It is generally accepted that blood pressure rises with age and it can also rise due to accidental damage in a local area. Here, we are looking at essential hypertension, the raising of blood pressure as we get older. As previously stated, we do not know for sure what is the actual cause of hypertension and why these phenomena affect us as we advance in years. Problems such as Diabetes also affect older people.

Why? Is it coincidental that diabetes and hypertension seem to be diagnosed in later life? It can be seen that it is very much in the interests of the health authorities to eliminate hypertension early in life, to ease the pressure on their finances in the future.

It has already been said that in times of stress the kidney produces Renin so blood pressure rises, however, we are not all under stress all the time, yet hypertension still occurs. Older people are likely to be under less stress than younger people are; yet still the older people are the ones who contract hypertension. So what is going on? According to my theory, as mentioned in chapter five, the heart pumps blood around the circulation system, aided by the brain, which through the nervous system causes the smooth muscle in the wall of the blood vessel to expand and hold open the vessels to their fullest diameter. The person is completely unaware of any such automatic actions being carried out by the brain in everyday life. As we grow older, it is reasonable to assume that everything is, to some degree, 'wearing out'.

This is also true of the neural distribution network. The system tires as a whole. This includes the filament nerves (the smallest in the body) which serve the blood vessels of the circulation system and carry the neuroflow from the brain to those blood vessels. This tiring effect is similar to the problem found in electrical work. Cables that have been terminated at electrical plugs are often left in the wall socket of an installation of a domestic house for years undisturbed. Let us consider an electric lamp that has been left plugged into the same wall socket for a long period of time. For some unapparent reason, the lamp can suddenly go out. When examined the plug is seen to have a perfect fuse but the cable connections to the plug terminals are broken in part or wholly. The reason is that cables carrying electrical current over many years simply wear out or become fatigued. The cable structure at the highly stressed point at which the cable is inserted into the screw terminal breaks and disconnects the electrical supply to the lamp. So, the cables wear out and as a result they are no longer able to allow electric current to pass through the plug to, in this case, the lamp, although the plug has been undisturbed for many years.

Nerves react in a similar way. Over a period of many years of life, active or otherwise, the use of the nervous system has been constantly transporting neuroflow. The wear and tear on the nervous system has been mounting, which means that the filament nerves leading to the blood vessels also tire. In effect, this will result in an impedance of neuroflow. The supply to the blood vessels is insufficient to maintain the full diameter of the artery or vein and consequently the wall of the blood vessel softens, and the pressure of the surrounding tissue or muscle reduces the cross sectional area of the tubes, the same as if it were a constriction. When this happens, all over the body, blood pressure begins to rise, slowly at first because it is a progressive event. Blood pressure (BP) climbs slowly. Usually this high BP reading is picked up at a much later date, perhaps at a health check, when the person is at about fifty years of age or so, by which time it may be too late. Now other organs in the body, which are designed to work with blood that arrives at a predetermined range of pressure, gradually find that the pressure is outside of their parameters. This may explain why some organs in the body give a lot of trouble after long term hypertension.

If a person has had all of their systems working correctly for the whole of their lives, then they can expect to have no trouble at all. For this to happen, the person's healing processes will have been quietly working away over the years. This ensures that neuroflow reaches every part of the body to its complete extent, guaranteeing that everything is working to the standard for that person, including the circulation system. It is true that some reduction of bodyweight is helpful where appropriate and where the genetic programme for an individual allows. This may lessen the shear volume of muscle and tissue, thus reducing the external pressure on the blood vessels. However, it is preferable to restore the neuroflow through the nerve network, thereby reinstating the integrity of the wall structure of the blood vessels. Losing weight will help but it is not getting to the root of the problem. We have seen above how it is that the blood pressure can rise over a number of years but is only detected later in life. By using Reflexology and experiencing the 'warmth' all over the body in a way that can be described as 'cosy', it can be interpreted that the healing plasma is healing and repairing the entire nerve network. Later, when the hands and feet actually feel warm what is being felt is the resumption of blood flow carrying with it full body heat. By this act, with the circulation system being as near fully restored as possible at this stage, the demand on the heart is reduced and it returns to a normal pattern of work, thus a more healthy situation is restored. This then is how I believe that blood pressure is caused and dealt with when the knowledge, as shown in this book, is comprehended and used.

To illustrate this further, I would like to recall the case of a seventy year old woman who came to my clinic. She had trouble walking around the town, having to stop and sit down at every other shop. Her back was giving a lot of pain. She had been asked to lose some weight by her doctor and this was proving very difficult. I commenced treatment for the complaint as previously stated in this book, but this time putting more emphasis on the spine, neck, shoulders, arms and sciatic nerve reflexes. She told me that she was hypertensive and was having medication, as prescribed by her doctor. After six weeks of Reflexology treatment, she reported that she could now walk into and around town, then walk home again, all without having to stop and rest. She was delighted. She confessed that she had feared becoming housebound. During those six weeks of treatment she would get very warm in the lower back and both legs. In addition to this, she would get quite warm all over her body. At the end of the Reflexology treatment, she would visit the toilet and then leave. After she had left, I sat and wondered about this. Why had she been so warm universally?

She arrived in the seventh week, told me that she had been to see the doctor, and asked if she could stop taking the painkillers that he had been prescribed. The doctor had said she could reduce the dosage and go back to see him in another four weeks. Meanwhile, the doctor measured her blood pressure with a sphygmomanometer and was pleased to see that her blood pressure had reduced a little. She told me that she was delighted. I gave her another treatment and she reported the warmth in her lower back which then spread to being warm all over her body. She was relaxed and after a short recovery time, she left. I was beginning to connect the universal warmth with the drop in her blood pressure. This seemed a reasonable thing to conclude because before she had started treatment, she had hypertension, but now she was having treatment the blood pressure was reducing. There seemed to be only one reasonable conclusion to be drawn.

Over the next four weeks she received the same treatment and experienced the same pattern of warmth. The following week she told me that the doctor had again measured her blood pressure and told her that it was down even more. By this time she had stopped taking the painkillers completely. In my opinion it was the Reflexology that had replaced her need for drugs of this type. She received Reflexology treatment and again she experienced the same warm feelings. This treatment pattern went on for four months, by which time her lower back was in good condition. She was due to see her doctor again after which she came back to see me with the good news that her blood pressure reading was normal. So she had asked if she could stop taking the pills for hypertension altogether. He said she should not cease taking them at the moment but go on reducing them slowly and he would review things again in six months. My client was now coming for regular treatment at agreed intervals. She attended the next appointment with the doctor with a certain amount of excitement. Her doctor measured her blood pressure again and found that it was still normal. He then agreed for her to come off the tablets for hypertension altogether. She was overjoyed.

There is no doubt in my mind that the healing process was going back over her entire nervous network and gradually restoring the condition to where it should be as determined by the individual's genetic blueprint. Thus it allowed the full neuroflow to affect the blood vessels and reduce the pressure in her system. Her feet and hands were now physically warm all the time. She had not lost any weight during this time but could now walk into town, walk round and walk home again without hindrance.

Chapter 10

The Hormonal System and Breast Cancer

For the most part hormones are produced by the endocrine system. The glands that make up this system are:
Pituitary - Thymus - Thyroid - Parathyroids - Adrenal Glands - Testes/ Ovaries - Prostrate/Uterus.
The whole subject of hormones is vast and cannot be dealt with here. What we will do is look at some of the implications of the ways in which they do or don't affect our lives.

Hormones are essential to life in both men and women. It is normally with women that we associate 'hormone' problems, indeed they have a much more complex hormonal system , so there is more to go wrong. Men too have a hormone system, but it is less complex than that of a woman. When the man's hormone system is out of balance he can suffer from many of the problems that a woman gets. Currently less attention is being paid to the male problem but it exists nonetheless. Sex hormones in a woman are steroidal hormones produced by the ovaries and they are called - Oestrogen and Progesterone. Sex hormones in a man are steroidal hormones produced by the testes and are called - Testosterone.

These hormones control the reproductive systems of both sexes and when the reproductive system produces less or an inadequate quantity of the 'standard' for the hormone system of an individual, things such as the menstrual cycle start to go wrong and problems such as mood swings appear. This is why doctors in some instances prescribe hormone replacement therapy (H.R.T). The idea is to replace the natural hormones that seem to be lacking in the body with an artificial replica. This treatment is available to both women and men but it is associated mostly with women. When women take H.R.T it is often said by the patients that they feel extremely well. This is to be expected because the medication has swamped the hormone system with a fixed amount of imported hormones. When this happens, all the difficulties that had been experienced by the individual have been corrected by the H.R.T. and cleared up. This puts the individual back to the standard and restores the person to their Lifepath. No wonder they feel good again.

I would not want to deny anyone the chance to feel good, but we must understand that the original maladjustment(s) that caused the problem in the first place is still there. As that symptom is put into the background and has been overwhelmed by the H.R.T it no longer causes the original difficulty, hence the person feels on top of the world. By taking H.R.T we are putting the body into a false dimension. The person feels great, but the original problem is still there, suppressed. The H.R.T has performed an operational change without doing anything about the reason for its requirement in the first instance.

I hear of people who have taken H.R.T then being advised by their doctor, for one reason or another, to cease taking it. This causes the body to be denied the quantity of hormone previously supplied and after a while the original problems come to the fore again. I have seen in some of my clients where, after stopping H.R.T the menstrual difficulties and resulting ailments, such as migraine or any panic feelings they previously suffered from, have all returned. It is entirely understandable that, faced with this situation, a woman will be tempted to continue with H.R.T rather than risk the surfacing of all the old problems again. It is therefore clear to me that the original ailments must be attended to so that the person can resume their own Lifepath back to normality, without the need for imported hormonal support. Women have come to my clinic with menstrual difficulties, such as irregularity in the monthly cycle, heavy bleeding and painful periods. Often they complain of migraines, anxiety feelings, panic attacks, lumps in the breast and mastitis. From my records I noticed that many women have one or more such problems but these are always linked with a difficult menstrual cycle. Sometimes these difficulties go back many years but always the menstrual periods were bad a long time before the subsequent complaints arose. Those women without any sign of a problem with the menstrual cycle did not appear to have any of the difficulties mentioned above. I concluded that if it were possible to give help in putting right the menstrual cycle, which must have been the standard for the person, the other apparently related problems would just disappear.

An example of this is a case where a woman came to my clinic complaining of large lumps in her breasts and heavy bleeding at menstruation. She had been told that there was nothing to worry about, but of course she was very worried. A friend of hers had referred her to me. The first week, having obtained, what I thought was the whole story, I proceeded to apply a complete treatment of Reflexology. After the main treatment was completed I went back and re-treated the reflexes for sacrum and coccyx, ovaries, uterus, sciatic nerves, sacro iliac joint, the whole of the spine, the autonomic system, both breasts and pituitary gland. This treatment initiated the healing process and she said she felt warm in the lower back, bottom, thighs and tummy; in fact everything between the waist line and the knees. In addition she had a 'hot' feeling in each breast. The warmth died down at the end of the treatment session, but she was very relaxed. I gave her some time to recover and she then left.

The second week she reported that she had felt 'terrible' and much worse than before. I surmised that we had obviously caused a change to take place in the hormone system and she agreed. The same treatment pattern was used that week and she reported the same feeling of warmth but not so much in the breasts. At the end of the session she felt relaxed and left. The third week arrived and she told me that she still had panic feelings. What panic feelings? These were unknown to me up until now, however things had started to settle down. On the fourth week she came to the clinic and said that her period had arrived but it was not so heavy as it usually was. The breast lumps remained and she still had feelings of panic, although not so intense.

The fifth week came around and she reported that she was feeling much better and her husband had noticed the improvement. Her panic feelings had left her. The breast lumps had changed shape and they were smaller than before. I gave her the same treatment for Reflexology as in the first week and all subsequent weeks. At the end of the session she reported that she could feel the warmth in both breasts as well as below the waist to the knees, including the tummy. She left after resting to recover. The sixth and seventh weeks were much the same as the fifth week.

The eighth week came and she reported that the period had arrived on time and was as normal as it could be. The lumps in the breasts were now almost gone. The same Reflexology treatment was given as in previous weeks. After the session, she felt warm in the breasts and in her lower back and tummy. Having recovered, she left in a good frame of mind. The ninth week arrived and she was looking as pleased as punch. She said that all lumps in her breasts had now gone but she was almost unwilling to talk about it for fear that they would return. The treatment had shown up the reflexes in the sciatic nerves only. Afterwards, she felt warmth only in her lower back, but faintly this time. She was delighted. On this occasion she did not need to recover; she was full of vitality.

The tenth week she called to see me we talked a lot about what had happened. I explained that in my opinion, Reflexology had persuaded her body to alter the hormonal balance in her body and had dealt with the situation on two fronts, gynaecological and via the brain. She had felt heat in the whole of her tummy and her lower back while the healing plasma was attending to the complete gynaecological system. If the brain cannot see that there is a problem, no specific treatment is given because it is not aware that there is problem to reverse. Maybe the ovaries go wrong and do not produce enough hormones for the healthy body. The lumps may have been corrected because of the same reason in that the connection from the brain to the breasts was impeded at the neck and once this impedance was removed healing plasma to each breast was increased and the lumps just disappeared. This would take her back to the standard for the operation of her systems and had restored her to the Lifepath. I explained that I thought the healing process had been working each week and that is why she had felt warm. The fact that she had felt warm in the area from the waistline to the knees initially was evidence to me that the healing process was attending to the reproductive system and her nerve system. This had caused a change in the way the system had been working and it was now back to where it should be. She agreed that she now felt better than she had done for many years and was more able to cope with her life. What was more, she no longer had to rely on drug therapy and that made her feel very happy indeed.

This woman had indeed experienced the enormous ability of the body to right itself, the natural way, with Reflexology being the catalyst. I thought it wise for her to return to me for treatment once a month which she did, but no lumps have returned to her breasts. During the course of the succeeding months, she has regarded the monthly treatments as preventative, however, we have been able to pick up other ailments that affected her, such as backache, and she is entirely happy with the situation. Due to her wonderful progress, we both agreed that she could now visit me every two months.

Lumps in the breast(s) can be alarming for a client. In view of the above, I have to conclude that lumps are the result of the menstrual cycle going wrong, perhaps due to a stiff or aching lower back and inflammation in the neck. When the cycle was put right the lumps just disappeared because the reason for their existence was no longer there. In my opinion, there is no other explanation. This is good news for a woman who now can correct in a simple way, many things that might trouble her, by using Reflexology. I would like to hazard a guess that this case could be recognised in many people. Does anything ring true for you? An imbalance in the hormone system can create havoc within a person. It really is worth getting a Reflexologist to do something about it. I have not seen any such example presented to me by a man, but I have no reason to doubt that if one did, the result would be just as rewarding. It might also be the case that many gynaecological problems can be resolved in this way.

Over the last two or three years I have been assailed by a flow of requests for money. These requests have been for the Cancer Research Campaign, Imperial Cancer Research Fund and now the World Cancer Research Fund. In addition there are local calls for money from friends of hospices and so on. Cancer is clearly exercising the minds of a vast number of people and I am full of admiration for those involved in this field of medicine.

No one seems to know precisely what causes cancer so we find that a variety of efforts are made in the hope that one or other will help. These efforts are to be applauded and supported. Most of the money raised goes into research and aftercare. The demands upon the nation's purse is unending and will eventually reach a plateau, from which funds will decline as pressure for funds in other areas increases. I get many people through my clinic with various problems, which is why I have set up a web site. The two things that new clients often ask are, "Can you do anything about Aids and Cancer?" Of course we do not know if we can, but it does not stop me from thinking about it.

About four years ago I saw a Panorama programme on television which highlighted the appalling discrepancy between the way in which various hospitals were using X-ray machines. The programme also featured graphics and I must assume that these were based on factual information. The viewer was shown the way in which the X-ray stream was not unlike a stream of water, it "feathered". We were told that the particles that feathered smashed through healthy tissue. There was a lot more, including an interview with the then head of the N.R.P.B (National Radiological Protection Board), who said that there was no safe dosage of X-ray emissions or of E.M.F (Electro-Magnetic Force).

This stayed in my mind for some years until I wrote this book on how Reflexology works. I started to think in the same investigative manner about cancer. I realised that there seems to be many forms of cancer, so I limited my thoughts to breast cancer and bowel cancer. My book describes in broad terms, how the body looks after itself and the essential 'rules' which are employed to allow this to happen. I assume that these 'rules' by which the body operates apply to both the good and the bad. In the case of breast cancer, I set about asking my clients who had contracted breast cancer or had a friend or relative who suffered with the disease, the chronological events that lead up to the diagnosis of cancer. There is nothing in the body that is specifically designed to do any harm to the individual, from which I exclude the acid in the stomach. If we accept this simple premise then something from outside the body has made the change. But what?

A woman has a complicated hormone structure and if her body is to function in the predetermined manner in which it should, it is necessary for a near perfect internal environment. This also means that the hormone producing areas in the body must function correctly. For this to happen, the brain, that is the centre of all intelligence, needs to monitor everything through the neural network so that it can initiate remedial action and repair if necessary. This allows the function to continue, as it should.

If the brain cannot monitor the state of the ovaries, for example, no remedial action can be taken and the ovaries change. This will result in an over or under production of hormones, and whichever way it happens, the result is an imbalance in the hormonal structure. Add to this the fact that should the patient have a neck problem and inflammation prevents the brain from seeing what is going on in the breast, then if a lump is being produced the brain cannot see what has gone wrong and therefore cannot initiate remedial action. This lump is the result of long term imbalance in the hormonal structure due to inflammation in the lower back and the neck. I have found this to be the case with all those I questioned, some thirty people. The lump should not be there at all and is a foreign material, even though the body produced it. Therefore the lump can be an unstable structure.

The chronological events that followed the discovery of the lump went as follows: lump discovered - visit to doctor - referred to hospital - X-ray ordered. It is my belief that at this point the lump is not malignant. The X-rays smash through the cell structure and break up some cells, but not all. The smashed cells with half of the D.N.A start to look for other cells to plug into and replicate. The result is the formation of any entirely different material and it spreads by replication. Stray half-cells that are aggressively looking for a home get taken up by the lymph fluid and taken to the nearest lymph node, which explains why, from a biopsy, it is sometimes hard to spot the cancerous cells because the biopsy happens to have been taken at a time when the cancer cells have not spread through the lump. There have been some occasions where it may even be that at the time of the biopsy the medic has missed the cancerous cells altogether. The patient is relieved but finds out later that the lump is changing shape and a subsequent visit to the hospital results in a positive biopsy and diagnosis: Cancer. It is my theory that the same applies to bowel cancer as to breast cancer because the rules of the body apply throughout.

I have had a few people tell me that my theories are not applicable. Here are some examples: A woman client was very happy to discuss her breast cancer and mastectomy. She had felt a lump in her breast and went to the doctor. A biopsy was taken, but no X-ray. She was promptly told that she had cancer. A little while later, she told me that she personally had not had an X-ray, but she had been around horses when they were being X-rayed. I asked what had actually happened at such an occasion and she explained that the vet and assistant stood on one side of the horse, fully clothed in protective gear, and placed the X-ray machine in front of them. My client stood on the other side of the horse and was given a protective apron up to the waist, which was to protect the ovaries. My client was present at more than one such event. She admitted that she was already aware she had a lump, but did nothing about it until it started to change. Originally she had come to me for long-standing back and neck pains, both of which had now subsided.

A woman told me about her husband who had died of cancer, and he had complained of severe back pain for years, and consequently had taken a technical job to allow him to sit more. He had had a lot of bowel 'trouble' for years, then began to suffer with severe tummy pain and was referred to hospital. There, a biopsy was taken and cancer was diagnosed. An operation was performed for the removal of the cancer, but he died soon afterwards. My client was quite content to talk about it and together we discussed my theory. She said that it could not be true because he had never had an X-ray. A little while later, she said that although he had not been X-rayed, he had worked in a small room nearby and was heavily involved with aerials and antennae and had worked a lot at close hand with microwaves. My theory appeared to still be holding up.

It is my opinion that there could be a correlation between the breast lump and X-ray examination. Currently, we use X-ray examination because this is the only way available to see what is going on inside the body. If this basic tool of medicine is at fault then we need to re-assess how we can achieve a similar function but by using less invasive methods. X-rays are used to produce a picture onto a photographic plate and this is accomplished by passing an irradiated stream through the body. If we look at the body as it is, we can see that it is made up of a variety of materials such as hair, skin, blood, muscle (of various types), bones and organic material. Each and every material has a different density and therefore retains and releases heat at an individual rate. It seems to be well within the capability of our technological industries that they construct a way to see this phenomenon. The basic approach is to detect the different heat/vibrational sources emanating from a body and pass this data to a computer. In this way and with suitable software, a perfect picture could be seen with no risk to the patient. Three dimensional pictures and moving pictures should also be possible. In this way, no invasive procedures are carried out which in my opinion may adversely influence any lump that may be present.

I have developed a new approach to Reflexology and call this Neuroflexology (R2 - Reflexology -at the second level). Using this method, I believe it may be possible to encourage the body to work on removing such lumps, before it becomes necessary to resort to surgery.

Osteoporosis
Definition: Oxford Reference Concise Medical Dictionary. 'Loss of boney tissue resulting in bones being brittle and liable to fracture. Infection, injury and synovitis can cause localised osteoporosis of an adjacent bone. Generalised osteoporosis is common in elderly people. Women often experience osteoporosis after the menopause. It is also a feature of Cushings disease and prolonged steroid therapy'.

The definition states that menopausal women often contract osteoporosis. It is highly likely that a woman with a poor menstrual life has an unbalanced hormone system and carries this imbalance into menopause. This is borne out by some of the women coming to my clinic. During and after the menopause, the reproductive system does not expire altogether, it merely slows right down so that ovulation cannot take place, but some hormone production carries on to keep the body healthy and in good working order.

For a man the less complex hormonal system and physical characteristics mean that he does not have a physical menopause. However, an imbalance in a man's hormonal system for many years may be the cause of some men contracting osteoporosis, in the same way that a woman does. Reflexology can help here but it should not be left until the problem is diagnosed. The earlier treatment can commence the more one can feel secure. In both cases, if the hormonal system has come through life in good shape then boney tissue should have been produced at the correct replacement level throughout that life. If the hormonal system has been upset and is not supplying the correct value of hormone necessary to sustain healthy boney tissue, then problems can be expected later in life, or after menopause for women. The result may well be deterioration of the bone density and osteoporosis. As I have shown above, by using Reflexology treatment much earlier in life the hormonal system may be restored, however it is unlikely that a reversal of the situation can be achieved after the diagnosis for osteoporosis has been made, but a holding situation may be possible.

In a woman, the ovaries need to be kept in good condition and normally this is the case. If the brain is in constant contact with the ovaries through the neural network, then they receive their full quota of healing plasma. If the neuro flow is impeded then the ovaries will not perform correctly. This may well happen because of inflammation in the lower back, and if the hormone production is adversely affected it is quite easy to see that bones will possibly lose some density because they need hormones to produce bone material. Similarly, if the imbalance of hormones persists, then, as hormones are used extensively in the brain, this may well affect the client's mind. It is therefore very important to keep the hormone levels in balance. In my opinion, just adding a synthetic hormone to the body will not do. I believe that the basic cause of the problem must be addressed and Reflexology can do this naturally.

It is recognised that not every woman who has a poor menstrual life gets osteoporosis. The degree of the problem will depend on the severity of the menstrual problem earlier in life. The body is the best judge of what it needs and what it can produce from within to defend and repair itself. We are inclined to forget that the body is designed to be self-sufficient, which means that we have the ability to keep away some of the nasty problems without additional intervention.

Chapter 11

Generally Speaking

Doctors are well trained people who go through much hardship to achieve their status. Their knowledge and perceptions are shaped along well defined lines, which have stood the test of time. One cannot and should not, place any doubt upon their pedigree and purpose. This does not mean that knowledge of medicine is totally confined within their ranks. The influence of Chinese medicine, which has developed along different lines, has gradually been taken more seriously in Western culture and perhaps this is a time for looking at alternative views and ways of achieving patient comfort. A different perspective may be all that is necessary.

A doctor, when presented with a patient's symptoms, will go down a familiar path of diagnosis and treatment as his/her training has directed. With the help of drugs and hospitals the recovery of the patient is their sole concern. Side effects of any drug are unwelcome for the patient, yet these abound. With Reflexology there are no such side effects because there is nothing given to the client to take.

Observations of clients during and after a Reflexology treatment have given cause to note that a set of happenings have been common to many. Each one has experienced 'warmth'. When Reflexologists talk about energy, I believe that this is the 'warmth' which their clients tell them about. I hope that I have shown here that this is not energy as most would understand the word, but the product of a perfectly natural physiological process. To understand the nature of this process is to further one's understanding of the body's integrity. Armed with the ability that this knowledge gives to one, a Reflexologist is enabled to help people more positively.

The warm or cosy feeling that people feel is an indication of the healing process, which is described elsewhere in this book. Where the client feels the cosy or general warmth, it indicates that following the Reflexology treatment the healing plasma has been circulated throughout the body. It coats the whole of the nerve network. Like an ointment, the healing plasma cleans and repairs each of the myriads of nerves . Once it has attended to these and has allowed the full neuroflow to be reinstated, the brain regains monitoring control of everything, including the blood supply system; increased oxygen, nutrients, body heat and products of the healing system can reach their proper targets. Each event will be accorded, perhaps not more but instead, the correct amount that enables the system to function within the parameters for which it was designed. This affects the muscles and organs, which all benefit from this vigorously reinstated supply once more.

When the blood carries body heat in the correct quantity to the extremities of the system, i.e. hands and feet, they too physically warm up. The healing process carries on usually without the knowledge of the client, quietly and without fuss. During a Reflexology treatment, all that I have described in this book occurs. The only indication to the client that anything different is happening is that they feel 'warm' all over and particularly warm in the area that was previously giving them trouble.

In the case of hypertension, it should be remembered that this explanation is applicable to the normal ageing process and makes no allowance for exceptional circumstances such as accidents. However, even then, the Lifepath dictates that the body must be returned to normality for the individual. When an accident causes damage to the body, the healing process (inflammatory process) immediately sets to work by restoring the systems allowing full neuroflow to stream. This gives back full control to the brain.

Because of the length of time that a problem may have existed it might not be possible for the body to recover as fully as would be desired after one treatment. Therefore a number of visits to a Reflexologist may well be necessary. Each visit is progressive, with the current treatment building on top of the previous one. This is because the amount of the healing plasma that the body can produce at any one time may not be sufficient to satisfy the problem completely. Instead several visits are necessary until the difficulty is overcome, and if the original problem seems to be resolved, the client is quite entitled to go back to the doctor and request a review of the medicinal regime that the doctor has initiated. This should be done with the declared requirement of the client that the drug therapy be stopped. The doctor must be satisfied, as must the client, that it is safe to do so.

In these pages it can be seen that if the theories hold good for arthritis and blood pressure, how much more could be affected by these theories. If a woman has gynaecological problems of any sort it could be that the inflammation in the lower back is blocking the brain's contact with the uterus. Could this be why women have to have D and C (Dilatation and Courettage) procedures, prolapses and even perhaps, why some people have miscarriages. It is all to do with impedance of information.

Chapter 12

Finally

I had thought that this might have been the end of my journey but instead I believe this is only the start of a much longer and greater journey. If this was the end, there would be no real point to the existence of this book, however its purpose is to stimulate ideas and further thought. If I had read such a book as this, I would be wondering what relevance with reality do these theories have? The answer is that these theories contain a great deal, if they are read with a sense of inquisitiveness. Those who say they "do not believe in it" seem to deny what is actually happening to them and it is only because these words have not come from a 'recognised' source that denial is preferred. Some do not want to acknowledge what is possible, some will refuse to think positively about this book because their whole training and background has taught them to see things in the way prescribed by their established and eminent predecessors, whilst others will never have given it a thought and regard the whole thing as 'hocus-pocus'.

I have written this book because it needed to be written. I have set out my thoughts and conclusions and it is my hope that you have enjoyed the journey with me thus far.

Appendix

The Future?

The future is full of hope and change. Change is the enemy of the establishment and fear is the result. We should not take fear from this book but rather seek how we can effect change for the improved health of nations and save money in the process.

After reading all that is written in this book you could be forgiven for thinking that you should go and see a Reflexologist. If you are a Reflexologist you might think that perhaps more training is required, or that you can't cope with the new thinking. To take the implications of what is written we could extrapolate the information and come up with a revolutionary scenario.

The State Health Service & Commercially Operated Health System

This is a service that can be divided into two parts, each one at loggerheads with the other.

1. The State Health Service is the service that cares for the health of the nation. Dedicated staff look on this as a vocation and many work the hours that most others outside the service would just not tolerate. It has a management side that is necessary to run the buildings, staff, drugs, surgery and beds and everyone in the industry feels some influence on the health structure of the nation. Nurses express worry over the mass of drugs they are asked to administer. In the case of commercially run healthcare the same applies, with a possible exception to the hours worked.

2. The financial side of the service. This applies to a state organised

and financially supported organisation. It also applies to a commercially operated system where a national service is carried out by commercially operated hospitals.

In almost every case there is conflict between the two parts. The one not being able to carry out what it sees as its duty in the manner thought most appropriate, and the other not having sufficient funds for this purpose and being branded by the other as being bureaucratic and expensive in itself and absorbing money that could be spent better on the care side of the service.

The care side of the service has, in recent years, seen an explosion in the need to bring in highly technical, innovative equipment. The cost of such equipment is escalating fast, even to the point at which, in the foreseeable future, only the richest hospitals will be able to budget for. It has seen the rise of specialist hospitals and the demise of local hospitals, and these latter establishments had previously been a great source of pride for urban and rural areas. Larger and more cost effective hospitals have been necessary to meet the need of the care and financial factions alike.

Here, I will attempt to show how such information as contained in this book could be put to good use for the benefit of the people and to combat financial constraints.

Imagine what it would like in a world where there was virtually no arthritis. What would that mean?

There would be no need for most hip and knee replacements, which would mean no more surgery for this purpose. Of course not all surgery would disappear, but probably some 90% would just not be required. This would apply to operating theatres and equipment associated with these procedures. The drug bill would be reduced and care would return to a local level.

Heart and circulation difficulties are emotive subjects and anything to do with them should be dealt with carefully. However, the plain fact is that the information contained in this book could well mean that at a guess, some 50% of expenditure on heart/circulation related illnesses could easily be cut.

It is possible that the intensive care units would largely be unnecessary if the number of heart cases was reduced.

Half the surgeons may not be required. Many kidney and liver operations could be eliminated and probably dialysis would be reduced.

Surgery to neck, arms and hands could be reduced dramatically. And so on…

The same thinking applied to general practice would have similar effects. The drug bill would probably drop by 50% or more and the GP could make good use of the local hospitals where, instead of going through expensive routes such as physiotherapy, pain clinics and consultants, they could attack peoples 'illnesses' at source and provide comfort without drugs, simply by implementing a radical change and providing Reflexology, or even better, NEUROFLEXOLOGY supported by the State.

Imagine what an enormous impact this would have financially. Of course, a great number of people would need to be trained in this new method of applying Reflexology, but the bill for all this would in no way match today's expenditure. The nurses affected by this rethink could be retrained and the existing Reflexologists could be brought into the scheme. I believe that we could lesson the cases of osteo-arthritic disease by 80%, reduce heart attacks by 50% or more within ten years, and much more besides. The ramifications of this are enormous. Could we dare to think it? A great leap of faith would be required but as the saying goes, faint heart never won fair maiden.

The one person we must not leave out is the client. Many people fear going into hospital but we will always need hospitals and specialists. Some say that people feel worse after having been in hospital. The method of treating people that I have developed and with the knowledge contained in this book, we would be able to free up the hospitals and GP's surgeries. We would start to really treat the client's problems in a far more cost effective and non-evasive way and would gain client approval. This may also overcome people's fears of the new super bugs that seem to be out-running our best antibiotic treatments. This would leave drug companies to get on with finding the real drugs to fight against real and external diseases.

If you have read this book and can correlate the content with your own experience, then perhaps the dawning of the truth can begin.

END

Neuroflexology

Neuroflexology – This is an upgrade on Reflexology and can be learned from the Internet – www.practalk.com/neuroflexology.html
Home web site – www.neuroflexology.com

Index

Rethinking Reflexology   by   John C F Moorhouse